MARY JANE

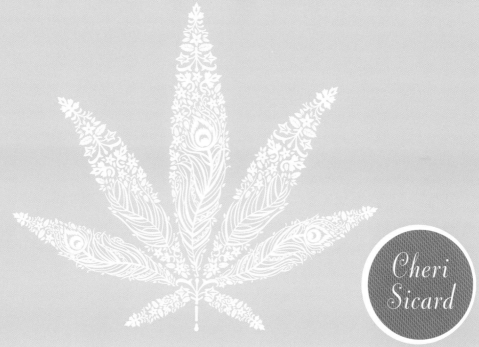

Cheri Sicard

THE COMPLETE MARIJUANA HANDBOOK *for* WOMEN

SEAL PRESS

CONTENTS

INTRODUCTION: On Women and Weed • 1

1 CANNABIS 101: The Grass That's Always Greener • 5

2 SMOKE SIGNALS AND VAPOR TRAILS: Inhaling Marijuana • 15

3 EXTRACTS WITH IMPACT: Hash, Wax, Oil, and Other Concentrates • 31

4 JOINT CUSTODY: How to Get Your Own Cannabis • 39

5 WEED THE PEOPLE: Know Your Rights • 49

6 PAGING DR. MARY JANE: Medical Marijuana • 59

7 YOGANJA! Healthy Living with Mary Jane • 71

8 FARMER JANE: Grow Your Own • 79

9 STIRRING THE POT: Cooking with Cannabis • 97

10 THE CANNA SUTRA: Buds in the Bedroom • 117

11 MARIJUANA MAMAS: Cannabis and Parenting • 125

12 HANDY HEMPY HOUSEHOLD HINTS: Pot Parties, DIY Projects, Keeping Your Green Clean, and More • 133

13 STARRING MARY JANE: Cannabis in Entertainment • 143

14 HOP ON THE CANNABUS: Traveling with Mary Jane • 169

15 KUSHY JOBS: Careers in the Cannabis Industry • 181

16 YES WE CANNABIS! Be an Open Advocate • 189

17 GET ON YOUR HIGH HORSE: How to Win Any Argument about Marijuana • 199

APPENDIX: Through the Years with Mary Jane: A Cannabis Chronology • 212

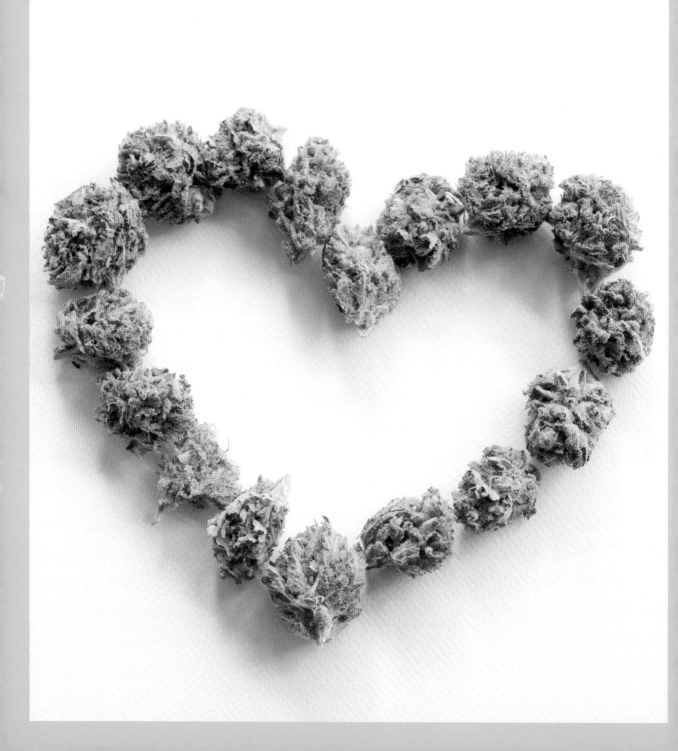

INTRODUCTION

on WOMEN and WEED

Turn on the news, read a magazine, or watch a television talk show these days and you are likely to encounter stories about "Marijuana Moms," who say the herb makes them better parents, "Stiletto Stoners," successful career women who prefer ganja to an after-work glass of wine or cocktail, or "Grandmas Smoking Pot" as a natural replacement for a host of pharmaceutical medications.

While these stereotypes are little more than clichés, they still tell us something important: The media are finally waking up to the fact that their longtime portrayal of the typical marijuana user as a male slacker who resembles Cheech and/or Chong is old school, outdated, and embarrassingly limited.

Until recently, men have dominated the world of cannabis, from the top master growers to the most vocal activists to the male-centric stoner rap music and stoner buddy comedy movies. This is pretty ironic when you consider the fact that marijuana itself is matriarchal. After all, it's only the prized flowers from female marijuana plants that we smoke, vaporize, or turn into concentrates or edibles. And you can bet if you overhear a marijuana grower talking about "the girls," he's not talking about his daughters or even referring to his wife's breasts, but rather his crop of female cannabis plants.

So why haven't more women been involved with this female-centric plant world before? The reasons are many—from social stigmas to fear to being misinformed about or unaware of the real, undisputable facts about marijuana.

I too used to be one of those uninformed people, and truthfully I didn't care—I believed that, because I didn't use marijuana, the issue did not affect me. As you will see in the pages ahead, I could not have been more wrong because the cannabis issue crosses over into so many others that marijuana legalization, or the lack thereof, affects everyone—regardless of whether or not they themselves ever actually light up.

I came late to this party. Other than the occasional puff at a party, I didn't use marijuana until I was almost forty. After a host of pharmaceutical and homeopathic remedies had failed, my doctor recommended I try cannabis for a chronic nausea problem. (He said it off the record because the HMO he worked for did not officially allow him to suggest this.) I tried it and it worked, immediately.

After a few months, I also noticed that the chronic gastrointestinal pain and discomfort that had plagued me since childhood had disappeared. I also no longer felt the need for my prescription antidepressants.

Because the public is beginning to understand the truth about this plant that corporate and government interests have tried to keep hidden since the 1930s, women are coming out of the Cannabis Closet like never before, and not just celebrities like Rihanna, Melissa Etheridge, and Jennifer Aniston (to name only a few) but ordinary women like your friends, neighbors, relatives, and perhaps even you! Just as they did when ending alcohol Prohibition, women are repeating history and making significant contributions to ending marijuana prohibition. These powerful, successful, and inspiring ladies have come to realize the war on cannabis does far more harm to their families and society at large than the substance ever could, even if all the reefer madness propaganda was taken at face value.

This book will be your guide to the wonderful world of weed—it will dispel the myths and misinformation you may have accepted as truth, and teach you how you can best incorporate marijuana into your life in a way that makes sense for *you*. I'll strip away the hype and sensationalism to give you the straight dope (pun intended!) on the science and insider culture of cannabis, and to answer the questions I'm asked over and over again on my blog and at speaking engagements and classes. In other words, expect this book to cover a spectrum of marijuana knowledge— from critical and potentially lifesaving to fun and frivolous.

Marijuana truly is the great equalizer. People who would otherwise have little to nothing in common have been known to connect and bond over cannabis, and in the process learn they actually have far more in common than they originally perceived. Just think what this could do on a global scale.

I'd like to buy the world a toke!

—*Cheri Sicard*

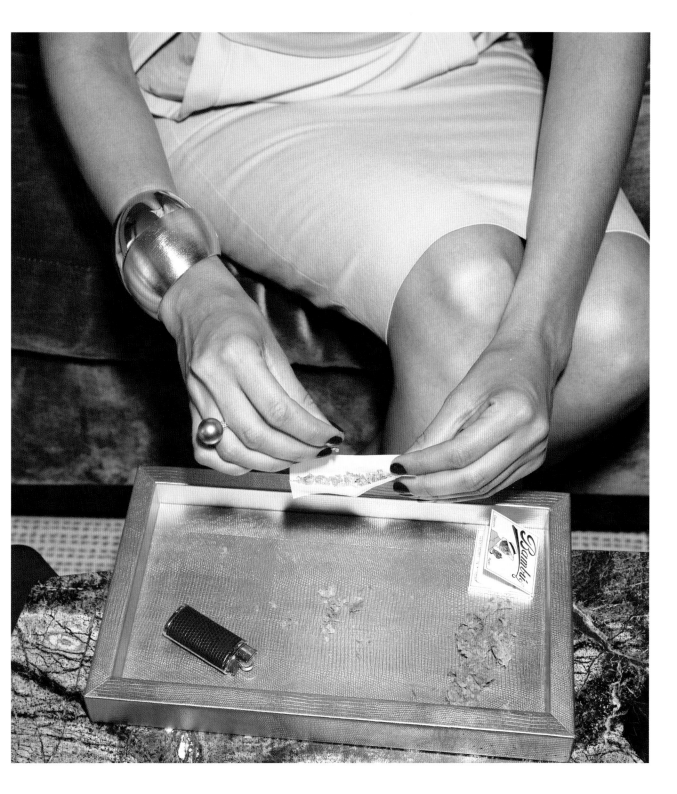

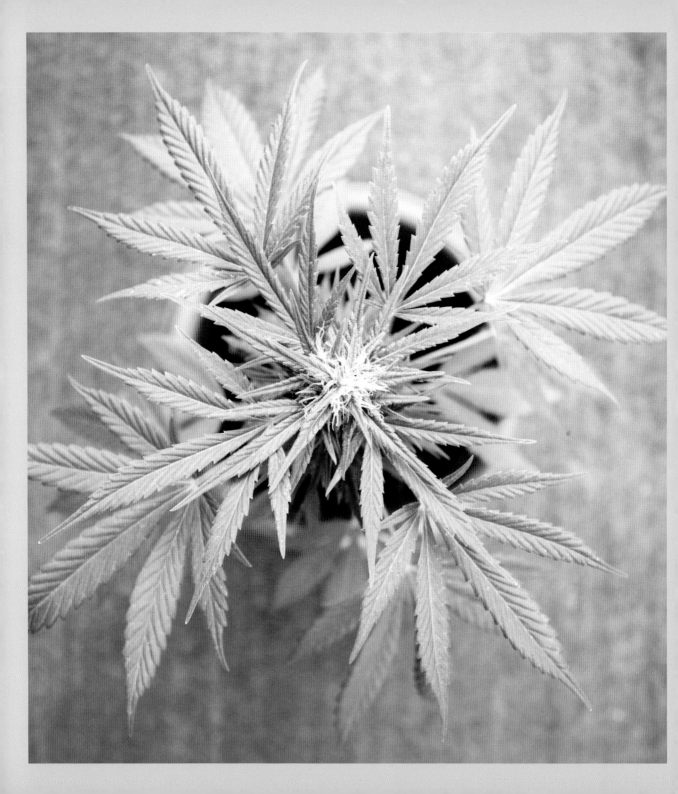

CHAPTER 1

CANNABIS 101:
the GRASS that's ALWAYS GREENER

Welcome to Mary Jane University, the very best place for your higher education! The very first step we must take is to get one important piece of information out in the open:

Marijuana is safe.

There has never, ever been a single death credibly attributed to marijuana overdose. It is virtually impossible to fatally overdose on weed. You could technically eat enough of it to burst your stomach or choke on it, and there were recent news reports of a South American man who was crushed under thousands of pounds of it, but that's about it.

The same goes for serious bodily damage in the form of organ failure. It simply does not work that way in the body. Unlike alcohol, many prescription drugs, and a lot of over-the-counter drugs, you are not going to damage your liver, kidneys, lungs, or brain, even with heavy use. And despite the government's dire warnings and Schedule I drug label, marijuana's most common side effects are nothing more than dry mouth and mild euphoria. For a nation that's addicted to anti-depressants, that doesn't sound like such a bad thing!

Now that's settled, let's get oriented in the world of weed! If you are lucky enough to live in a state that has legalized marijuana for medicinal and/or recreational use, the days of buying seed-filled, hard-as-a-brick-and-dry-as-a-desert-marijuana are gone. Cannabis options have become so sophisticated! Quality indicas, sativas, hybrids—not to mention a head-spinning array of cannabis strains with wild names like Headband, Strawberry Cough, Sour Diesel, and Girl Scout Cookies—await shoppers at clean, brightly lit marijuana shops.

However, for those who live in states where marijuana remains completely illegal, buyers have to deal with less cultured options, generally called *schwag* (see page 7 for more on this). But be aware, change is coming everywhere. And soon. And when it does, you will be ready, wherever you live! Let's get started!

GETTING ACQUAINTED WITH STRAINS: INDICAS, SATIVAS, AND HYBRIDS

Thousands of individual marijuana strains exist, each with subtle and sometimes not so subtle differences, but virtually all marijuana can be categorized as one of three types: indica, sativa, or hybrid. I say "virtually" because another type exists (*Cannabis ruderalis*), but the average consumer will likely never encounter this wild-growing subspecies.

You might think of these three categories as the marijuana equivalent of red, white, and blush in wines, under which you can find countless variations. As with wine, some people have a definite preference for one or the other. Most connoisseurs, however, like both, at various occasions and times for various reasons.

While both sativa and indica varieties of *Cannabis Sativa* (I know, the semantics are confusing) have medicinal properties and both will get you high, there are important differences between the two.

Cannabis Sativa

Plant appearance: Long, tall, thin plants with narrow leaves.

Origins: Southeast Asia, Mexico, Colombia, Thailand.

Effects: Energetic, euphoric, mood-lifting, creative head high.

Medical treatment: Relieves stress, depression, and nausea; stimulates appetite.

Possible downside: Strong sativas can make some people feel anxious or paranoid.

Cannabis Indica

Plant appearance: Shorter, stockier, and denser than sativas with broader leaves.

Origins: Afghanistan, Morocco, Tibet.

Effects: Relaxing body high.

Medical treatment: Relieves chronic pain, muscle spasms, and insomnia.

Possible downside: Strong indicas can induce what is known as "couch-lock," the state of being so stoned you have zero motivation to move from the sofa.

Many marijuana users are fond of saying, "Sativas will get you high; indicas will get you stoned." At times you may prefer one effect to the other, but more often than not you will want a little of both.

Enter the *hybrid*.

Nowadays you'll rarely find a pure indica or a pure sativa strain; most are in fact hybrids, giving users and growers the best qualities of both. In this third category, hybrids, the variations are endless. The mix might be evenly split between indica and sativa, or 60–40, or 70–30. You get the picture. Once you are familiar with how different strains work for you, you'll be able to choose strains based on their genetics.

Of course, you don't have to get nearly so refined. You can just smoke what's available, enjoy it, have a good time, and leave concern about varieties to others! Either way, now that you know the strains of cannabis, here are a few more common terms to know. They're a little more slang-like, but key to choosing the pot that's right for you:

Schwag (usually used as a noun but occasionally as an adjective) is the general term for cheap, low-quality marijuana. When someone mentions schwag, they usually mean dry, compacted weed filled with seeds, stems, and a lot of leaf material, although it can refer to low-grade marijuana in general.

Dank (usually used as an adjective but occasionally as a noun) means the good stuff. It's green, sticky, fragrant, seedless, and potent. If someone tells you they procured some dank weed, you are definitely going to want to hit that (the weed, not the person)!

THE BUZZ:

CANNABIS VERSUS HEMP

Are cannabis and hemp the same thing? It can get confusing because the terms have often been used interchangeably. It is true that both come from the same plant, *Cannabis sativa*. However, hemp, or industrialized hemp, contains about 0.3–1.5 percent THC (the intoxicating component that makes you feel high), whereas marijuana typically contains 3–10 percent or more. Despite the federal government's uninformed claims, you will NOT get high smoking hemp. But you can make over 25,000 products from it!

Throughout this book, unless otherwise noted, hemp refers to the non-psychoactive cousin of cannabis or marijuana.

Sinsemilla (sin-seh-mee-ya, noun or adjective), from the Spanish for "without seeds," is a general term that refers to highly potent, seedless marijuana cultivated from unpollinated female plants. Pretty much anything you get from a reputable dispensary will be sinsemilla.

Shake refers to the broken pieces of buds that are at the bottom of a large bag of marijuana. Think of it as the cannabis equivalent of the crumbs at the bottom of a potato chip bag. Because consumers like big buds, dispensaries and dealers often sell shake at greatly reduced prices, so it can make a great way to get lower cost weed.

CRAZY ABOUT CANNABINOIDS

What exactly is cannabis made of? Cannabis contains more than sixty active chemicals, collectively known as *cannabinoids*, which are responsible for its medicinal effects. *Cannabinoids* are unique to this plant. They are not found anywhere else in nature . . . except in the bodies of living creatures!

That's right. All living creatures higher than mollusks on the evolutionary scale have an *endocannabinoid* system (lots more about this in Chapter 6) that produces natural or *endo*cannabinoids. What this means in practical terms is that each and every one of us is physiologically programmed to respond to cannabis. That's why cannabis works so well— it's perfectly suited to work with the chemistry in our own bodies.

In the documentary *What If Cannabis Cured Cancer?* Dr. Raphael Mechoulam, the Israeli scientist who first isolated THC, says the fact that we have a plant that mimics the body's natural endocannabinoids is "just a quirk of nature." Some quirk!

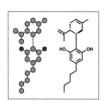

Cannabidiol (CBD) cannabis molecule

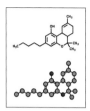

THC (delta-9-tetrahydro-cannabinol, dronabinol) cannabis drug molecule

CAN YOUR CANNABIS PASS THE TEST? HOW TO READ THE LABELS

As legal commercial marijuana markets emerge with the coming end of prohibition, laboratory-tested cannabis and cannabis products are becoming the industry standard. Some legal ordinances are already in place in areas of the country that require lab testing. But even where they aren't, leading industry providers have started providing this service as a matter of quality control and professionalism.

Not all lab tests are created equal, but good ones provide you with enough information to help you make smart choices. The levels of THC and CBD in each strain will give you an idea of how much marijuana you will need to smoke, vaporize, or eat in order to feel the effect. This is especially important with edibles because without this type of labeling it is impossible to know how much you are ingesting (not that ingesting too much is dangerous; uncomfortable perhaps, but not dangerous). Lab testing also makes sure the product is pure, free of mold, bacteria, and pesticides. Dr. Jeffrey Raber, director of the Werc Shop, one of the world's preeminent testing labs, says that over 25 percent of randomly tested products are contaminated, even more so with cannabis concentrates like waxes and oils. Raber told me that contamination with pesticides might not pose an immediate problem, but over time toxins can build up in the liver and kidneys.

The Werc Shop has published work in the *Journal of Toxicology* showing that up to 70 percent of the pesticides present on dried flower material can be transferred to the consumer via inhalation, a good argument for the consumer to grow or buy organic marijuana.

Since not all labs are as experienced or as thorough as the Werc Shop, look for clues that you're dealing with a good one. Labels that tell you the date when the product was tested assure you that what you are getting in the package actually matches what is on the label. Some providers have been known to cut corners by testing a given strain or batch of marijuana-infused edibles once and then

THE BUZZ:

THC AND HEAT

Delta-9-tetrahydrocannabinol, or THC, is the cannabinoid that gets all the publicity because it's the component that's responsible for making you feel high. What most people don't realize is that it doesn't even exist in the raw plant. That's right, eating raw marijuana will not make you high! Adding heat causes decarboxylation, a chemical reaction that converts the raw plant's THC-A (or acid) into the psychoactive substance THC.

assuming that the numbers will apply to all future crops and batches. This is obviously not accurate, especially if different growers cultivated their plants under different conditions.

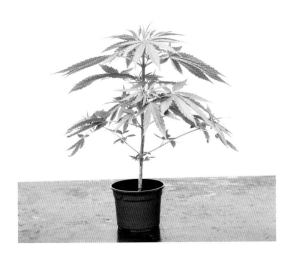

A young Cannabis Indica plant

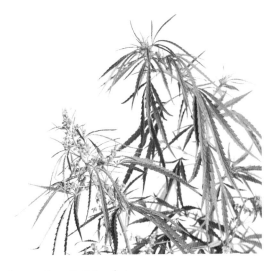

A mature Cannabis Sativa plant

WHAT'S WITH ALL THOSE CRAZY NAMES?

Sour Diesel, Headband, Strawberry Cough, Blue Dream, Luke Skywalker, Master Yoda, Rolling Thunder, Train Wreck, Jack the Ripper, Purple Urkle, Swerdlow OG—marijuana names have some pretty wild monikers, and these are some of the more polite ones.

The names have actually been around since the 1960s, when Maui Wowie, Panama Red, and Thai Sticks were all the rage, but with the proliferation of medical marijuana and legalization, this type of "branding" has grown like weeds (pun intended).

Connoisseurs well versed in cannabis genetics can sometimes glean clues from the strain names. For instance, I recently procured some fine Cherry Dream grown from seeds produced by master grower and breeder Kyle Kushman. Those in the know can decipher that this strain was born by crossing Blue Dream with Cherry Lopez. More often than not, though, the name has no greater significance than the whim of the person naming it. In many cases that person has a "Beavis and Butthead" level sense of humor.

Cannabis activists bemoan the fact that some of the more offensive strain names, such as Green Crack, God's Pussy, or Donkey Dick, hurt the movement, as they make it impossible to sell the concept of marijuana as serious medicine. They've got a point. But until this infant industry sorts itself out, and arguably even well after, we are stuck with crazy strain names. One plus, however, is that it does make it easier to remember your favorites.

MARIJUANA TASTING NOTES

You'll benefit from keeping some notes on your favorite strains. Think of yourself as a wine connoisseur who keeps tasting notes. Only replace the "wine" with "weed." Indicate the strain name, how it looked, smelled, and tasted, along with its potency and how it made you feel. Why all the physical descriptions? Because less ethical dispensaries or dealers may say you are getting certain strains when they really have no idea what the strain actually is. If you suspect that to be

MARIJUANA
FRESH BUDS

Sativa

Afghan

White widow

Hash

Silver haze

Morroccan

Dutch

White shark

Cheese

Hindu Kush

Skunk

Bubblegum

Caramel

PREMIUM QUALITY

Indica

• BEST IN TOWN •

ANATOMY OF A MARIJUANA PLANT
Essential Terms

Buds or *flowers* (the terms can be used interchangeably) are the dense buds of the plant. Covered in resinous glands known as *trichomes* that store the THC acid that will covert to THC upon decarboxylation, flowers represent the prime cuts of the cannabis world.

Tiny trichome-covered *sugar leaves* surround the buds. Some people like to leave these leaves intact and smoke or vape them along with the flowers (a bit harsher but still trichome-rich if they come from good plants). Sinsemilla snobs want only the buds, and most dispensary marijuana will be free from any leaves. Sugar leaves also make terrific hash (see Chapter 3) or cannabis-infused butter or oil (see Chapter 9).

If you don't grow your own, you'll never see *fan leaves*. While pretty, the ratio of plant materials to trichomes is too high to provide a good smoke. These leaves do have some trichomes, however, and can be used to make lesser grades of hash or in cooking.

You'll be a sad stoner when you get down to *seeds* and *stems* (they're never called twigs). Seeds are rare to nonexistent these days in good weed unless the plant was bred for that purpose, but common in *schwag*. If you do happen to find a seed or two in a batch of weed you like, put them aside and turn to Chapter 8.

the case, you can always compare your notes with a reputable book like the *Big Book of Buds* or an online reference and make sure you are getting what you expect. It's important, however, to note that that the same strain from a different grower or grown under different conditions will vary, especially in potency.

If you are using cannabis to treat specific medical conditions, there are practical reasons to keep notes because certain ailments respond better to certain strains. Because everyone's body chemistry is different, what works for your sister-in-law may not work best for you. Notes will help you keep track of how your condition(s) did or did not respond to different strains.

Notes will also allow you to refer back to favorite varieties in order to compare and contrast in the future. Trust me. There are so many different strains on the market these days that, even without the short-term memory loss marijuana is alleged to induce, it would be impossible to recall them all, much less the subtleties of how they affected you.

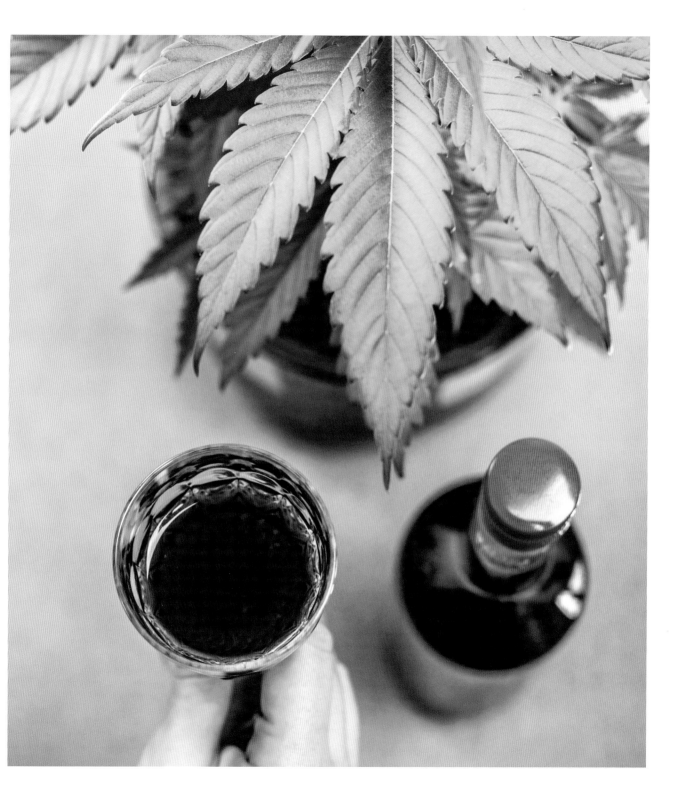

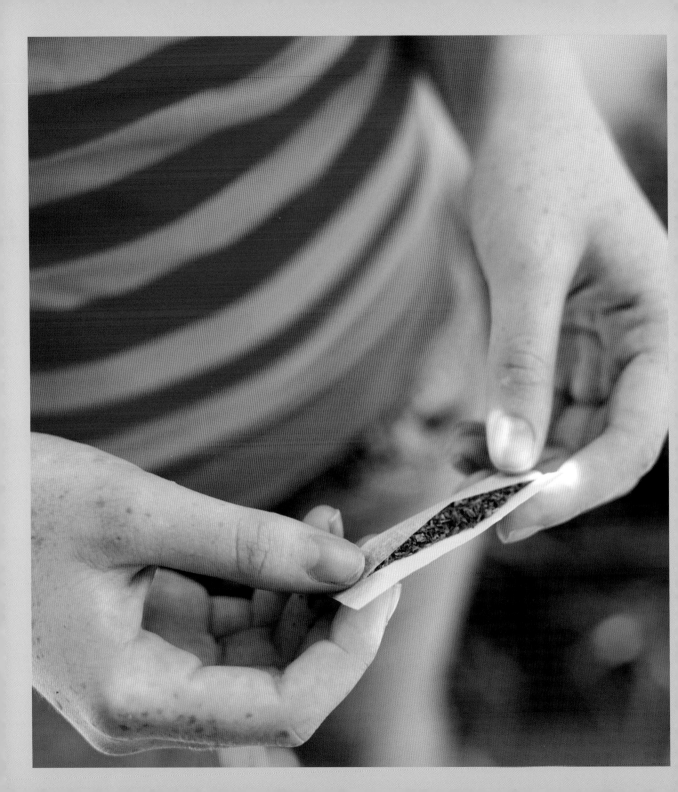

CHAPTER 2

SMOKE SIGNALS *and* VAPOR TRAILS: INHALING MARIJUANA

If you think smoking a joint, or a marijuana cigarette, is the only way to ingest cannabis, this chapter will open a whole new world for you. As cannabis is moving into the mainstream culture and more consumers are becoming interested in marijuana, an enormous array of pipes, bongs, one hitters, and vaporizers are exploding on the market. From party-sized accessories to individual vapor pen electronic "cigarettes," the ways to enjoy your weed have multiplied at a dizzying rate.

Every year brings better mousetraps. Attend any consumer cannabis expo or industry trade show and you'll find some amazing and innovative products that belong in the collections of most marijuana aficionados. You'll also find gadgets that will make you wonder what their inventors were smoking when they came up with that ridiculous idea.

In addition to the wide variety of equipment that helps you inhale marijuana, new consumer products will appeal to marijuana fans of every age and ilk. It is no longer necessary to smoke or even vaporize at all! Edible products of all kinds (see Chapter 9), topicals, and even transdermal patches can now deliver the benefits of cannabis with zero heat, smoke, vapor, or odor involved. Sometimes even without the high. (Yes, Virginia, some people actually do not want to get high.)

JOINT ASSETS

Before we explore other ingestion options, let's start with the aforementioned humble joint, or marijuana cigarette. It's a classic for a good reason: Joints are inexpensive, easy to carry and smoke, disposable, and sharable. On the downside, they do create a lot of smoke and aroma, so discreet they're not. If you're going to roll your own, here are some basics to know from the start:

- Grind your ganja. Grind or break up your plant material so it has an even consistency, and then remove any small stem pieces. (See "Gotta Have It! Grinders" for more.)

- Roll moderately. You want the finished joint to be firm enough that it will not fall apart or burn too fast, but not so tightly wound that it is impossible to inhale through.

- Pick proper papers. Go to any smoke shop and you'll find an enormous selection of rolling papers. Use the right size for the joint you are rolling—burning paper produces tar and does nothing to get you high, so you don't need any excess. Consider using a hemp or rice paper to keep the smoke all-natural.

- Place the plant material evenly along the length of your rolling paper's fold.

- Pick the whole thing up and start rolling back and forth, from the middle to the edges, keeping the plant material evenly distributed. According to one of my coleaders in the NORML Women's Alliance, if you roll from the middle, the edges will follow and you'll have a nice even joint instead of a pregnant worm.

- Once you are happy with the size and consistency of the marijuana cylinder, start rolling the excess paper around it. Lick the glue strip, seal that baby up, and you are ready to blaze!

Rolling joints takes a certain amount of practice and skill. Some people pick it up right away. Others go through years of producing joints that resemble a snake that just consumed a gerbil. But if you know how to roll by hand, you will always be prepared in a pinch. Get good at it and you might even win some prizes at joint-rolling contests. And with enough practice, you'll soon pick up speed and skill.

Your other option is to use a gadget. Even though I am the "Queen of Green," I still can't roll a decent joint by hand. The reason? I haven't practiced enough. (Who has the time?) It doesn't matter if you can't either because for about three bucks you can buy a simple little gadget called a "cigarette" roller, which will help you roll perfect joints, quickly and easily. Every time. "Cigarette" rollers keep everything nice and even. Put in the plant material, roll it up, insert paper, roll again, seal the glue strip, and you are done! They even come in different sizes to fit different rolling papers.

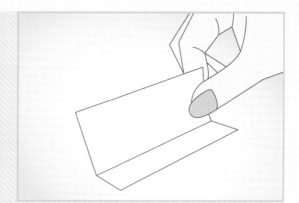

How to Roll a Joint

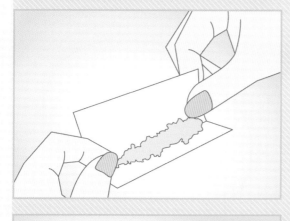

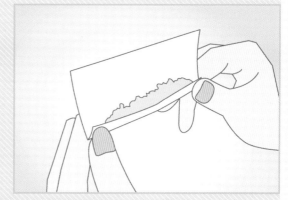

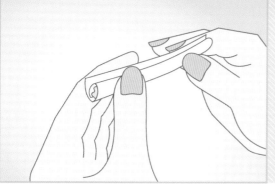

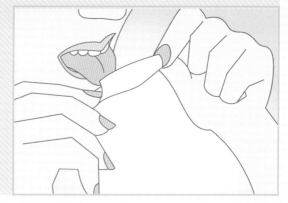

A JOINT BY ANY OTHER NAME IS STILL AS DANK

For such a simple item, the marijuana cigarette goes by many names and has inspired some interesting spin-offs. Here are the essential joint-related terms every *toker* (one who *tokes* or takes *hits* of marijuana) should know:

- *Joint, J, jay,* and **doobie** all refer to a simple marijuana cigarette.

- A **pre-roll** is simply a joint that you purchase rolled and ready to smoke from a marijuana dispensary or dealer.

- A **fatty, big fatty,** or **fat boy** is a large joint rolled with extra marijuana; conversely, a **pinner** is a thin, tightly rolled version of the same.

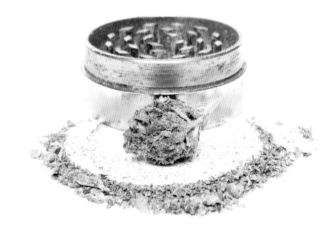

- A *blunt* or *dutchie* is a joint rolled in a tobacco leaf wrapper, like a cigar, instead of paper. A *spliff* refers to a joint of cannabis mixed with tobacco.

- You'll know you are in a *hotbox* situation when you find yourself in a closed space with one or more pot smokers who are filling the room with smoke from one or more joints. Since it has nowhere to escape, the exhaled smoke hangs in the air and gets re-inhaled for maximum effects. The word can also be used as a verb, as in "Wanda and Catrina hotboxed me in Jeff's van." (I know, it sounds sexual, but it's not.)

- In the marijuana world, *roaches* are a good thing! This term refers to the smoked down butt of a joint. Thrifty folk can extend their *stash*, or supply of marijuana, by saving roaches, taking them apart, removing the paper, and combining what's left—known as *roach weed*. Put it in a pipe or roll another joint and enjoy!

- When it comes to joints, you don't want to eat the *cherry*, or red burning end, but you do want to hit it right away or you will be wasting weed.

- And finally, when someone tells you that your joint *has a run* or is *running*, that means it is burning unevenly, with one vertical side being smoked down to ash and the other remaining stubbornly intact. A run in a joint sort of resembles a run in a stocking. Stop a joint from running by applying a spot of saliva or water to the paper just beneath the run and relight.

PIPE DREAMS

Pipes come in every imaginable size, shape, style, and price. They range from simple to sophisticated, and everything in between. Add to that the fact that almost ANYTHING can be turned into a pipe (see Chapter 12) and you've got endless possibilities.

- *Glass* burns clean, and there is a huge variety to choose from. Depending on your taste, budget, and lifestyle, glass pipes can range from simple, functional workhorses to prestigious art pieces and stoner status symbols. The downside is that glass pipes can be fragile and, depending on size and design, can get hot.

- *Metal* pipes are inexpensive and durable, but, if you're not careful, the fast-moving heat can burn your lips.

OOOOH, THAT SMELL!

While I love the aroma of marijuana, there are any number of occasions when a girl needs to be discreet—say, around non-toking friends or family, when kids are nearby, in a nonsmoking hotel, or any time you are transporting marijuana in a car or in public. Here are some odor control tips:

- If you are worried about carrying marijuana on your person because of the smell (see Chapter 4), know that flowers have a far stronger fragrance than hash, oils, wax, tinctures, or edibles. Carry accordingly.

- Joints are by far the smokiest and smelliest of ingestion methods. Avoid them if you need to be discreet. Air freshener isn't much help and burning incense is almost as clear a signal as smoking weed itself.

- Vaporizers, conversely, are the most discreet way to inhale. The odor is slight at best and evaporates almost instantly.

- A low-tech stoner trick is to make a *spoof*, or portable filter, out of an empty cardboard tube—toilet paper tube, aluminum foil tube, paper towel tube, or any kind of tube you can get your hands on. Use elastic bands to secure a scented dryer fabric softener sheet over each end of the tube. Exhale the smoke directly through a dryer sheet and into the tube to filter out the smell. It's not 100 percent, but it does help a lot, provided you don't take too many back-to-back hits and you change the filters every now and then.

- Even better than a spoof is the Smoke Buddy, a personal air filter. Blow smoke in one end and the built-in carbon filter turns it into clean odorless air before it comes out the other end. (It works for tobacco too.) Genius! See www.smokebuddy.com.

- Putting a towel under the door helps to contain scents in one room until they fully dissipate.

- While artificial scents like air fresheners aren't always effective, you can sometimes overpower a moderate cannabis scent with enough other strong scents: think roasting garlic on the savory side or simmering cinnamon, ginger, and cloves on the sweet side. Or diffuse fragrant essential oils like lavender or citrus in simmering water.

- **Wood** is natural and durable, and it does not retain or conduct heat. It can, however, be difficult to clean.

- **Stone** is natural, like wood, and somewhat durable. But it can get very hot and may break if dropped.

BONGS

A bong is a pipe in which the smoke gets filtered through water before it gets to your lungs, in theory making for a cooler, smoother smoke. The number of styles, sizes, and types of bongs rivals pipes, from cheap, lightweight acrylic models to elaborate glass art pieces.

People can get extreme about their bongs. You might have seen bongs that are so comically long you need to stand on a ladder if you want to smoke from them. There are also delicate multi-chambered glass pieces that cost a fortune and can shatter into a million pieces with one false move. There are even ice bongs that allow you to freeze the water container to supposedly render a cooler smoke. It's debatable whether the temperature of the water makes much difference, but you can get the same effect by adding ice cubes to any bong water.

Speaking of bong water, change it often—I suggest you change the water with each new smoking session—and take care to never spill it. Spilled bong water has a pungent smoky stench that lingers long after the water itself is gone.

When buying a bong, consider how you are going to use it. Will it be an everyday thing or only for special occasions? If the latter, why not go a little more wild? But for everyday use, choose something that's sturdy, so it won't break or spill and that is easy to clean.

PIPE AND BONG LINGO

Let's bring you up to speed on the language of pipes and bongs so you can understand the conversation.

A **carburetor**, or **carb** for short, is a small air hole on a pipe or bong. Not all smoking implements have carbs, but, when they do, you will want to cover the hole with your finger as you begin to inhale and then let go at the last second in order to let all the smoke in the pipe or bong flow into your lungs. In lieu of a carb, some bongs have removable bowls that lift out at the end of the hit to allow you to inhale all the smoke in the tube.

One hitters are pipes designed to deliver a single hit (or two small hits). They are best for when you are out and about and need to discreetly sneak away for a puff. The many varieties all share the common denominator of small size. Some one hitters are also **sneak-a-tokes** or **stealth pipes**; in other words, they

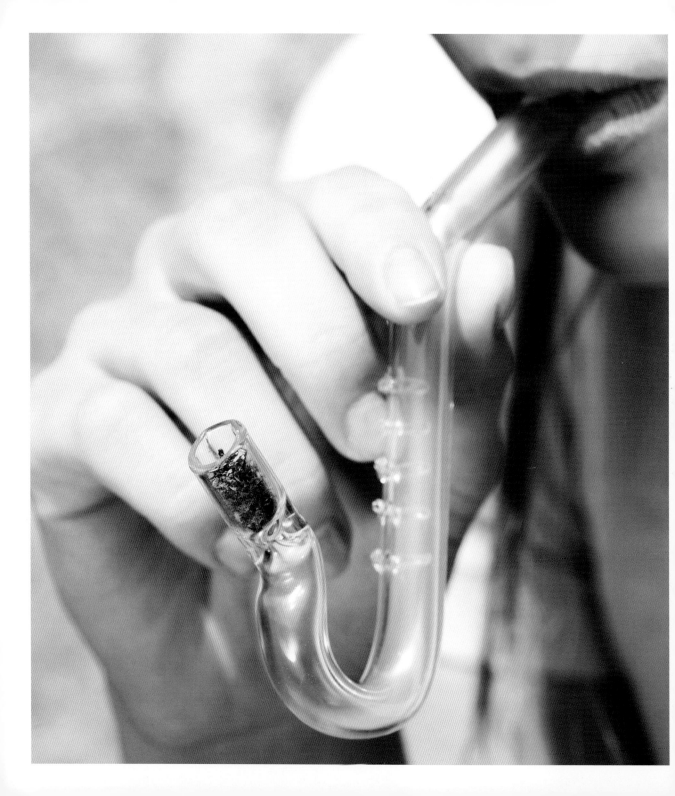

may not look like pipes at all. One popular variety looks like ordinary cigarettes (except they are made of metal or ceramic). James Bond would be proud of some of the creative stealth pipes that resemble lipstick or cigars or hide a one hitter inside an ordinary ink pen, magic marker, or hemp bracelet.

A *dugout* is a discreet smoking kit that comes in a small box. It holds plant material and a small pipe, often one of the aforementioned cigarette imposters. Insert the pipe into the container and "dig out" a hit of marijuana.

Not ready to commit to a bong? A *bubbler pipe* is a small, inexpensive version that holds just a few tablespoons of water to filter the smoke.

A *hookah* is a Middle Eastern water pipe that usually has multiple smoking mouthpieces so that several people can smoke at once.

Essential smoking accessories include small round *screens* to prevent smokers from sucking in ash and plant material through the pipe, and *pokers* for poking through sediment, ash, and leftover resins after smoking.

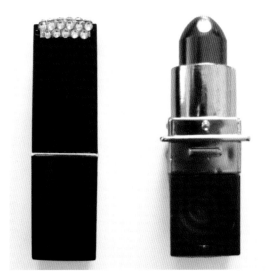

▲ *This stealth pipe is cleverly disguised as a lipstick*

And lest you sound uncool, know that you *hit a pipe* or *take a hit* off a pipe and *rip a bong* or *take a bong rip.*

VAPORIZING: A BETTER WAY TO INHALE

Many people do not want to smoke anything. At all. If you fall into this camp, don't confuse smoking with *vaping*—there's a difference.

The diaphanous cloud coming out of the mouth of someone who has just used a vaporizer might look like smoke, but it's not. Vaporizers turn the active ingredients in your marijuana into an inhalable vapor without actually combusting it. The vapor and the smell dissipate almost instantly.

Vaporizing used to be something known only to diehard stoners, but the dawn of medical and legalized marijuana has brought vaping into the mainstream—for tobacco smokers as well as marijuana users. The market is now flooded with vaporizers of every shape, size, style, and price point. Some allow you to vaporize plant material, whereas others use only concentrated oils and waxes. Some are versatile enough to use plants and/or oils and waxes.

When you smoke marijuana, you are inhaling not only the active ingredients— THC and other cannabinoids—but also the burning plant matter. And we know that smoke contains tar and carcinogens. Even though marijuana smoke does not cause lung cancer (see page 27), a survey by the Kaiser Permanente Center showed a 19 percent higher incidence of respiratory complaints among daily marijuana-only smokers than among nonsmokers.

Because the oil in cannabis can be vaporized at a lower temperature than it can be smoked, more THC and other cannabinoids are preserved. That's right, more bang for your buck! When you smoke marijuana, either flowers or concentrates, some of the THC and other cannabinoids burn away before they ever get into your lungs.

Without the taste of smoke, you'll also be able to more fully appreciate the flavor nuances of the cannabis. Expect a cleaner, more pronounced high.

Ideal Vaporizer Temperatures

Some vaporizers come with temperature controls. If yours doesn't, don't worry about it, but, if it does, pay attention. California NORML (National Organization for Reform of Marijuana Laws) cosponsored a study with MAPS (the Multi-Disciplinary Association for Psychedelic Studies) and found that vaporizers optimally produce THC at a temperature of 365 degrees Fahrenheit (185 degrees Celsius), although traces were in evidence at temperatures as low as 284 degrees F (140 degrees C).

NO BOGARTING!

The Etiquette of Smoking

Smoking marijuana is, by nature, a sociable and gracious activity. If you're smoking with others, always be generous, and familiarize yourself with these dos and don'ts:

Bogarting, the act of holding onto the pipe, joint, bong, or vaporizer bag—instead of passing to others—bears the name of the late actor Humphrey Bogart because he is frequently depicted with a cigarette hanging from his lips that he never appeared to smoke.

Puff, puff, pass is always the rule of the day in social smoking situations. The one exception is if you are, or even suspect you might be, getting sick. In that case you should carry and use your own personal smoking implement but still share your weed with the group as if you were passing, as they should share with you.

A song from British band Musical Youth advises us to "Pass the Dutchie on the Left-Hand Side." I've never known anyone to get hung up on this rule and have seen marijuana being passed to the left *and* right. You'll know you are at a good pot party when they come at you from both directions at once and getting rid of a joint becomes much like a game of hot potato. That said, if you find yourself at a loss about where to pass, to the left hand is always a good default position to fall back on.

However, don't pass a pipe that is *cashed*, or at minimum warn the next person in line of its depleted condition.

Becoming known for breaches of marijuana etiquette can come back to haunt you even decades later, as in the case of our *Bogarter* in Chief, who according to biographer David Maraniss in *Barack Obama: The Story*, was known in his pot-smoking high school days for *intercepting*, or cutting in line to take an extra pull, as the pipes or joints were passed.

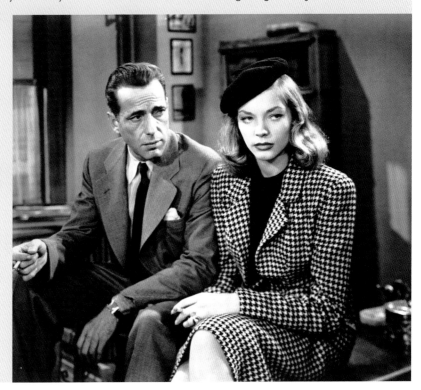

They also found that significant amounts of benzene, a known carcinogen, begin to appear at temperatures of 392 degrees F (200 degrees C). Whatever you do, resist the typical stoner frat boy urge to set your vaporizer at 420 degrees F. That's way too high!

So Many Vapes!

There are so many different vaporizers: electric, battery-charged, butane; vaporizers for flowers, hash, and/or oil—it would be impossible to cover all the variations, so let's start with the three most common types of vaporizers.

VAPE PENS

Today's pen-style vaporizers are virtually indistinguishable from electronic tobacco cigarettes. I'll let you draw your own conclusions about the advantage of that. A rechargeable lithium battery powers most of these portable personal vaporizers, which work best for vaporizing cannabis concentrate oils (see Chapter 3). Depending on the model, oil is loaded into the vaporizer or into a cartridge that is then loaded into the vaporizer. The oil will last for fifty hits or more—up to several hundred—depending on the brand of vaporizer.

Some companies claim that their pen vapes work with flowers. None of the brands I have tried have worked particularly well for this purpose, but new and better products come out all the time. My prediction is that, by the time this book comes out, this type of vape will have improved significantly.

As more and more brands have entered the marketplace, the price of vape pens has come down, way down. A vape pen used to cost several hundred dollars, but I have seen some at cannabis expos for as low as thirty bucks. Those didn't even make it through the after party. The same company in China manufactures products for many of the brand labels, but you still get what you pay for. When shopping around, look for clear instructions; a lot of brands come with sketchy half-English instructions at best. Never try to vape flowers or hash in a vape pen meant only for oil, or you'll clog the mechanism and render it useless. If you buy a vape pen that seems sturdy and comes from a known company with a reputable guarantee, you'll be on your way to a successful long-term relationship with your vaporizer pen.

TUBE STYLE

Under this broad heading, in which the vapor is inhaled via a clear plastic tube attached to the bowl—the part of the vaporizer that actually holds the plant material—you'll find many styles. Electricity, batteries, or even butane can power these vapes.

Simple, user-friendly box-style vaporizers consist of a small box that contains the

SHOCKING! MARIJUANA SMOKING NOT LINKED TO LUNG CANCER

It seems like common sense to think that smoking marijuana poses a lung cancer risk. After all, tobacco cigarettes irrefutably do, and marijuana smoke contains even more tar and carcinogens.

That's what Dr. Donald Tashkin and his team of UCLA researchers set out to prove once and for all. What they found shocked them and the medical community. After studying 2,000 actual human beings (not lab animals) over a period of ten years, they found no increase in the risk of developing lung cancer for marijuana smokers. Even heavy, long-term marijuana users who had smoked more than 20,000 joints over their lifetimes saw no increased lung cancer risk.

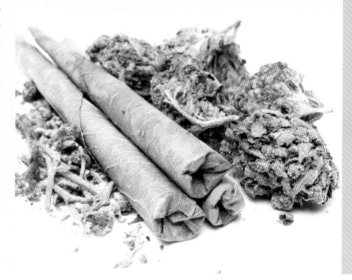

Tashkin did find that the more tobacco a subject smoked, the greater were his or her chances of developing lung cancer, but not so with cannabis. In fact, the tobacco smokers who also smoked marijuana had a slightly lower incidence of lung cancer than those who smoked tobacco alone.

Other studies of cannabis smoke and pulmonary function indicate that chronic exposure might be associated with an increased risk of certain respiratory complications, including a cough, bronchitis, and phlegm. However, ingesting cannabis via alternative methods (vaporizers, tinctures, or edibles) eliminates these issues.

heating element. Other handheld tube vaporizers, meant for home as well as travel use, contain everything in a more portable unit, about the size of a small milk carton. You get three to five hits out of most tube-style vaporizers before having to reload the bowl with fresh cannabis.

BALLOON STYLE

Balloon vaporizers work by pumping vaporized cannabis into a special balloon. Once full, the balloon is detached from the vaporizer, and the attached mouthpiece lets you take a draw anytime until the bag is empty. This offers the convenience of filling the bag and shutting off the vape, while having a ready-to-inhale supply of vaporized cannabis prepared.

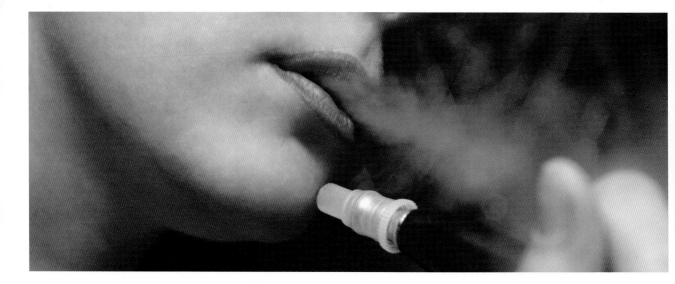

Bags come in all sizes too, from one that will hold a handful of hits to a huge party size that can be passed around a large group.

Expect to pay more for balloon vaporizers. They start at several hundred dollars and go up to over a thousand dollars. I have tried brands at various points on the price spectrum, and all have worked well. The difference lies in the specific features offered by each brand, including the guarantee. If you spend hundreds of dollars on a piece of vaporizing equipment, you want to know that the company who made it stands behind it. Volcano Brand sets the standard for this type of vaporizer to the point that the name is almost synonymous with the product, much as Kleenex is with tissues.

Stretching Your Stash: Vaporizer Leftovers

After smoking marijuana you are left with ash, making it obvious that it's cashed. Not so with vaporizing, when you are left with intact plant material. So how do you know when you need to load a new bowl? The exact cutoff point is partly a matter of personal taste, but you will notice the flavor take on some toasty notes. The color will also dull to dark green to greenish brown.

Some folks like to cook with the *duff*, or weed that's left after vaporizing—yes, there are still *some* cannabinoids left, as there are in flowers that have been *kiefed* (see Chapter 3). You'll need to use at least twice as much, but if you are on a tight budget, duff brownies beat nothing. If marijuana is plentiful in your world, you won't want to bother.

▸ *Cannabis bud surrounded by sugar leaves and fan leaves*

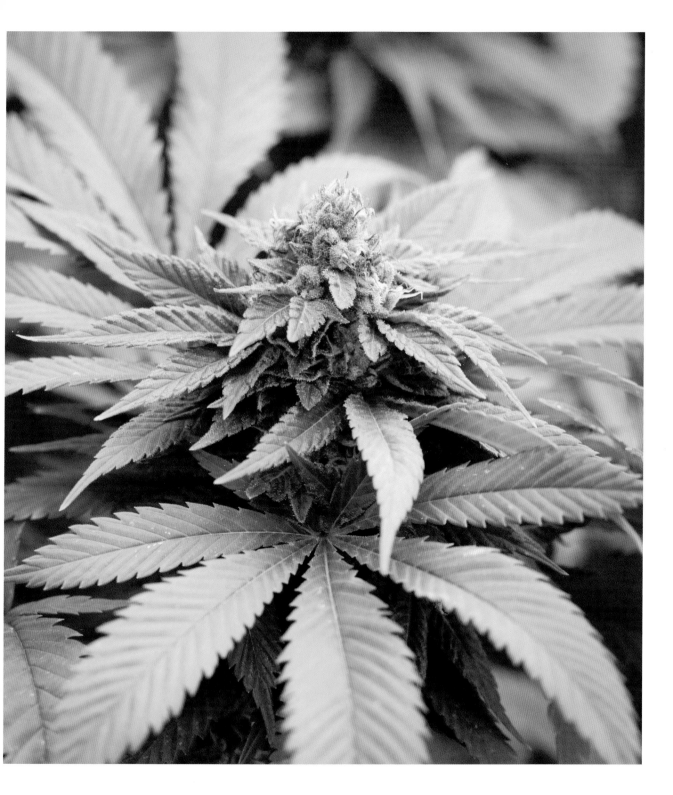

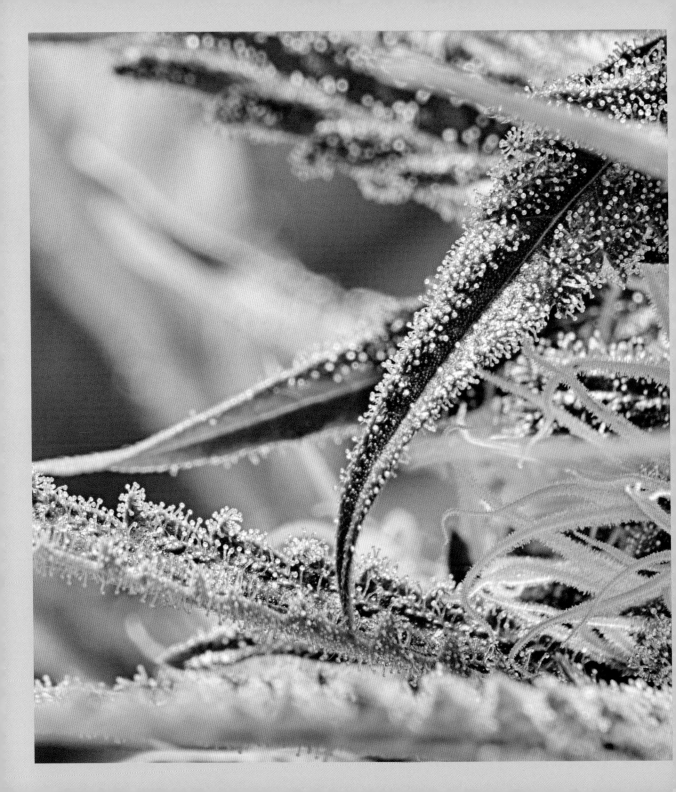

CHAPTER 3

EXTRACTS *with* IMPACT: HASH, WAX, OIL, *and* OTHER CONCENTRATES

Smoking is only one way to get your Mary Jane on. If you'd like to branch out and try something different, consider a concentrate. A cannabis concentrate refers to any product containing only the essential materials—the resinous glands, or trichomes, that cover the leaves and buds of marijuana plants—but having little to no actual plant material.

Some people like concentrates so much they use them exclusively. Others like to use them as well as buds. Here are some of the best qualities of concentrates:

- They are, well . . . concentrated, meaning you don't need to use much to get a proper dose. Those who need extra-strong doses can use them to up their cannabinoid intake to the level they need to treat their medical conditions.

- They are versatile—you can smoke, vaporize, and eat/cook with concentrates.

- They are discreet. A small amount of hash, oil, or wax concentrates can last far longer and take up less space in your purse or luggage than the equivalent in flowers. Concentrates also have less odor than the whole plant, both when carrying the product and ingesting it. In fact, today's vaporizer pens (see Chapter 2) are indistinguishable from electronic cigarettes and the slight aroma of the exhaled vapor evaporates instantly.

◀ *Trichomes on an immature cannabis plant. The clear trichomes will turn milky white and then amber as the plant matures*

- They can be economical. If you are growing your own, you can use trimmings and small trichome-covered "sugar leaves" that would otherwise be discarded to make concentrates.

- They can help make weak weed more potent. If you ever find yourself with marijuana whose potency is lacking, just augment it with concentrates. Sprinkle a little kief or dab on a little oil before smoking or vaping.

- They can help fine-tune effects. If you have a strong indica but you don't want to get couch-locked, you could help mitigate the effects by adding some sativa concentrate to your smoking or vaping mix, or vice versa.

Let's explore the most popular forms of marijuana concentrates you are likely to encounter, from the most natural and uncontroversial (if there is such a thing when talking about marijuana) all the way up to the King Kong of concentrates, Dabs.

Kief (pronounced "keef") refers to the sticky, resinous, THC-filled glands or trichomes that cover the cannabis plant. If you have ever noticed a fine powder at the bottom of a container of marijuana, you have seen kief. It can be smoked, vaporized, or used in cooking. For the latter, make sure heat is added to the mix; kief has not been decarboxylized, and, without the addition of heat, it won't get you high. Many marijuana grinders (see Chapter 2) come with built-in kief screens and chambers for collecting the kief.

Hash is kief, collected with either a wet or dry method, that has been heated and pressed. Depending on the plant material used, cannabis strain, and skill level of the person making it, hash can range from a dry, hard wafer that will need to be ground to a powder to a dense substance like sticky putty.

Water hash, sometimes also simply known as *hash*) is made by an all-natural water extraction process. Plant material, either flowers and/or trimmings, are agitated with ice water, which causes the resinous trichomes to become brittle and break off from the plant. The plant material is removed and the remaining water is strained through a series of increasingly smaller micron mesh filters. What remains is kief that is then pressed into hash of varying degrees of quality. Water hash is the easiest and least expensive concentrate, aside from kief, for the average home consumer to make. It's also the safest, regarding both the potential for physical danger and legal consequences because no chemicals are involved. Water hash can be smoked, vaporized, or used in cooking.

▶ *Honey oil aka Butane Hash Oil aka BHO*

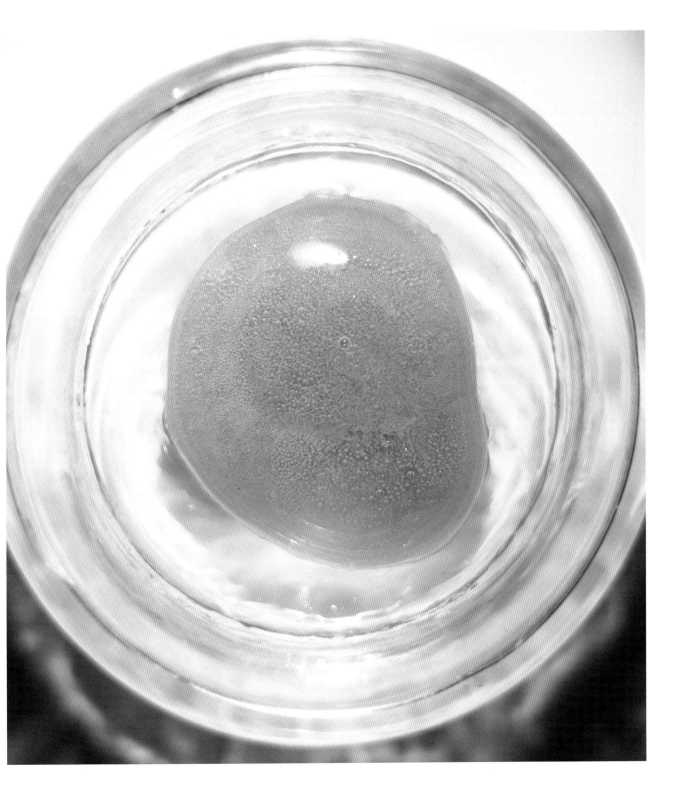

With the advent of medical marijuana, the medicine that was in nearly every American medicine cabinet in the 1930s has returned. *Tinctures,* infusions of cannabis in alcohol or glycerin, can be taken sublingually—just a few drops under the tongue—or added to foods.

Honey oil, wax, ear wax, and *shatter* are all concentrates of varying consistencies and thicknesses that have usually been made with a butane solvent extraction process. Likewise, these oils sometimes go under the collective label of BHO (butane hash oil). To make this product, the solvent is blasted through the plant material, which removes the trichomes, and then the solvent evaporates—most often with help from the *extraction artist.*

A public safety controversy arises because the process of making the oil or wax can lead to explosions and fires if not properly conducted and if the area where the concentrates are being made is not well ventilated.

If the solvent used wasn't pure or the plant material contained contaminants, chemical compounds can sometimes be left behind. Some people also worry about inhaling residual amounts of leftover solvent, which can happen if the concentrate wasn't sufficiently evaporated or *purged.*

As the legal cannabis industry grows, pure *critical extraction oils* are destined to become the standard. They are made in the same way as other herbal essential oils, using a carbon

dioxide extraction process and sophisticated equipment, which yields a clean (providing the plant material was clean), potent product. Critical extraction oils can be smoked, vaporized, or used in edibles.

Also known as *Rick Simpson Oil* or *RSO* (see sidebar), *Phoenix Tears* refers to a dark concentrate about the consistency of liquid tar, made by a simple chemical extraction method and low heat.

A LITTLE DAB'LL DO YA

Dabbing is, without a doubt, the hottest trend in cannabis today, especially with the twenty-something set, and especially in areas of the country where marijuana is legal or quasi-legal. The term comes from the act of placing a "dab" of wax or other similar BHO on a red hot metal (usually titanium) or glass nail.

When the dab hits the heat, it vaporizes. The imbiber inhales this vapor, usually through a sophisticated glass bong, and instantly gets seriously stoned.

It's been around for a decade or more, becoming trendy in Southern California but quickly spreading to other areas as easy access to cannabis concentrates expands.

Attend the High Times Cannabis Cup in California, Colorado, or Washington state and you will see people walking around with large, elaborate glass pipes and big butane torches. With all their equipment and paraphernalia, they are the stoner equivalent of those guys in the 1970s who carried enormous boom box stereos everywhere. These folks are die-hard dabbers equipped for a day of fun.

News organizations continually trot out fear-inducing stories about the dangers of dabbing and warn people about this new "craze." The meth-like paraphernalia typically used by dabbers (described above) has fueled a lot of the stories, and in fact it even makes a lot of long-term cannabis users uncomfortable.

Elaborate glassware and torches aside, when all is said and done, imbibers are still inhaling cannabis, which is still fundamentally safe even when highly concentrated.

To be sure, the negative dabbing stories might have some validity when it comes to the unknown element—the heated metal nail—that was added to the equation. Also, too much concentrated dabbing can result in severe throat irritation. It's also easy to overdo it and feel dizzy and disoriented. Take it easy, cowgirls, know your limits, dab with caution, and know that, even if you overdo it, the feeling should soon pass, unless you have other medical conditions that might be exacerbated by dabbing.

Safety Patrol: A Beginner's Guide to Dabbing

If you have never dabbed before, and especially if you consider yourself a cannabis lightweight, take some care if you decide to try dabbing. Here's how to make it a good experience:

- Have a seat. A dab hit comes on quickly and intensely. If you are not used to it, you may feel a little dizzy for a few seconds. Sit down to take the hit and stay there until you feel stable.

- Start small. A tiny dab is all you need. Dabs are HIGHLY concentrated, so it doesn't take a lot.

- Inhale carefully; exhale immediately. BHO vapor is expansive, meaning it is easy to get too big a hit, which will leave you coughing uncontrollably for some time afterward. And that's not fun. Or

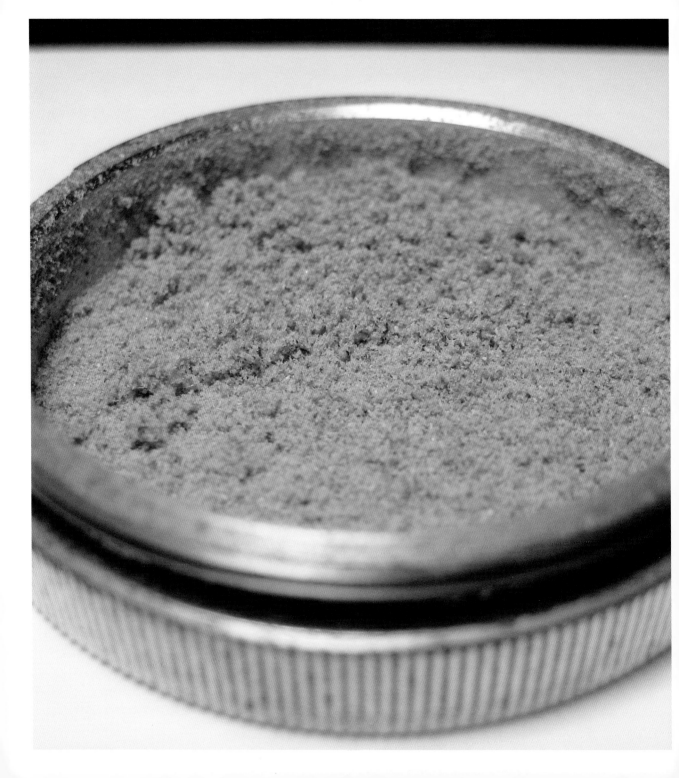

RICK SIMPSON:

Controversial Homespun Cannabis Hero

A few people might use Rick Simpson Oil recreationally, but most use it for serious medical conditions. It has not been scientifically tested, but there is an enormous amount of anecdotal evidence that RSO cures cancer and other serious ailments. It is named for Canadian Rick Simpson, who didn't invent the process but helped it gain international attention when he cured his own skin cancer with the oil. Nobody was more shocked than Simpson himself when doctors and government officials had no interest in his "miracle cure." Undeterred, Simpson continued making the oil and curing his friends and acquaintances, and the stories started to spread.

According to Dr. Jeffrey Raber of the Werc Shop (one of the world's leading testing laboratories), the major difference between RSO and other solvent extract concentrates is how they are made. Raber says solvents like hexane, naphtha, or isopropanol—chemicals that should not be ingested—are used in the extraction process for RSO (also called Phoenix Tears). Although all the solvents should have evaporated out of the final product, the Werc Shop has indeed found octane and even benzene, a known carcinogen, in some of the Phoenix Tears samples it has tested.

Today an Internet search for Rick Simpson Oil or Phoenix Tears yields scores of anecdotal stories from people who say their cancer was cured, along with detailed instructions on how to make the oil. You'll also find some skeptics disputing the claims. Until the end of prohibition opens the way for more medical research, it's doubtful that we'll know the specifics of Phoenix Tears, but science has already shown without a doubt that cannabis can kill cancer cells (see Chapter 6).

The documentary *Run from the Cure* (2008) chronicles the whole fascinating story of how Simpson came to use this medicine along with his quest to make cannabis therapy available to all, despite the legal and bureaucratic obstacles blocking his way.

ladylike. Take a smaller hit than you would when smoking flowers to allow for this difference. And you don't need to hold it either. Inhale and immediately start to slowly exhale (you don't need to hold it when smoking flowers either). It's better to do two small hits if you need to—and you probably won't—than one big one.

- Don't drive. You are going to feel a dab hit far more profoundly than the smoked or vaped equivalent in buds. Designate a driver or allow plenty of time for the effects to wear off before getting behind the wheel.

◀ *Grinder with a kief-catching receptacle*

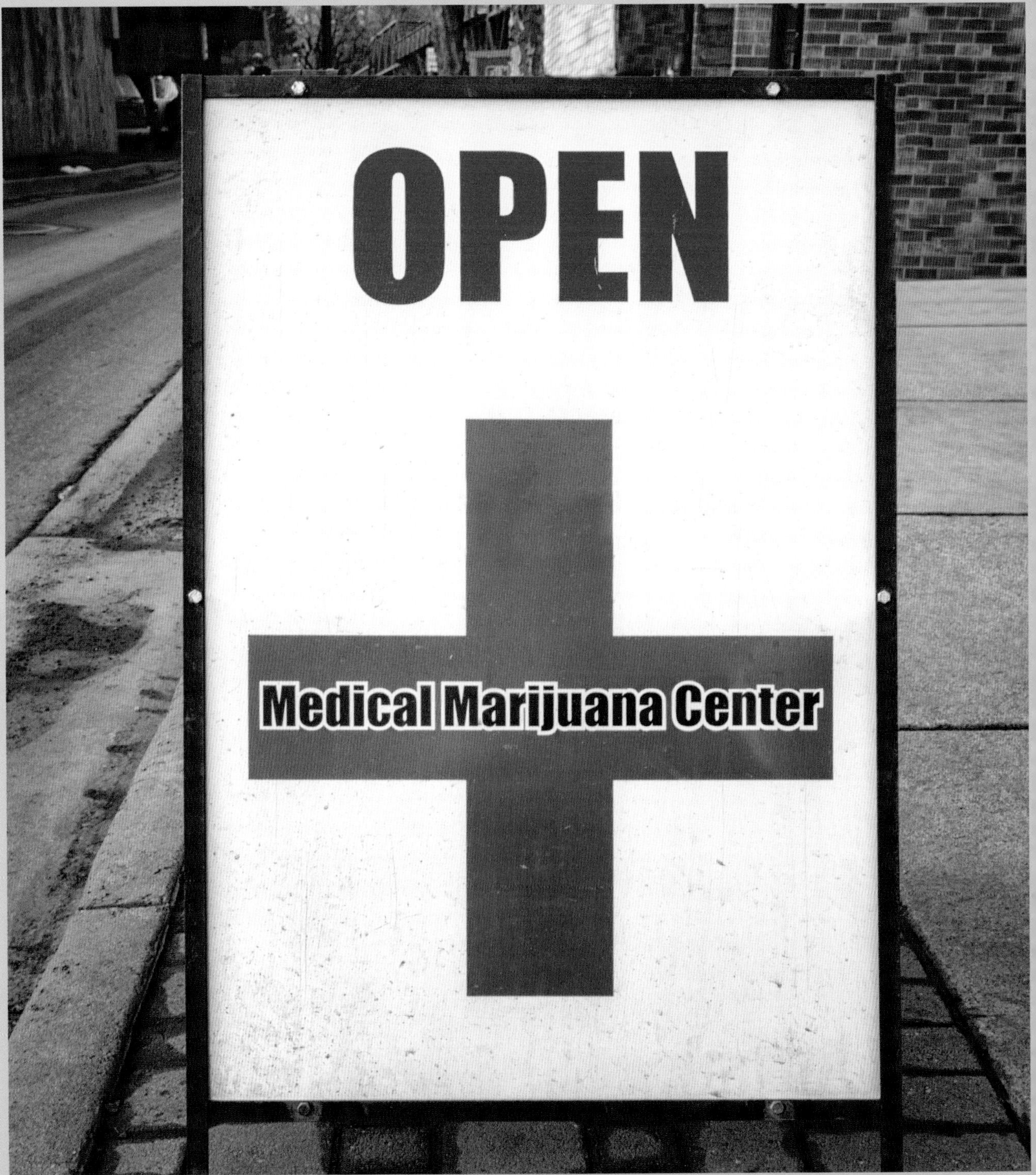
OPEN
Medical Marijuana Center

CHAPTER 4

JOINT CUSTODY:
HOW *to get* YOUR OWN CANNABIS

Procuring marijuana can be a big, time-consuming hassle, and even dangerous. Unless you grow your own or are lucky enough to know someone who does, where you obtain your marijuana will have a lot to do with where you live. In some cities and states you can just go to the store or have it delivered right to your door. In others, some unofficial form of buying is the only option. And in ALL scenarios, marijuana remains illegal at the federal level, so there is always some risk involved.

BUYING MARIJUANA WITHOUT A DISPENSARY

If you have a good source for buying cannabis, treat her well and keep her as long as you can. If not, you'll have to go on the hunt. Finding a hookup person—aka an "HP"—works best through friends. It's highly likely

you know someone who knows someone who can hook you up. Even if your friends are straight-laced, don't assume they don't indulge—the people who are regular pot smokers behind closed doors might shock you. You can test the waters by innocently bringing up the subject in conversation. Not a day goes by without marijuana being in the news (if you have trouble finding such stories, subscribe to my blog or follow me on Facebook). Pick a story, any story, and start a conversation about it to see how your friend reacts. You might also make a 420 joke or reference. If your friend chuckles, take the conversation to the next level; if you get a blank stare, move on. (If you yourself are staring blankly now, learn more about 420 in Chapter 14).

Here are some more suggestions to help you root out an acquaintance or two who might be sympathetic to your plight, or make some new friends whose interests are more in line with your own.

The person you are talking to just might be a stoner if . . .

- there's always incense burning in her home;

- she often has red eyes;

- she always carries a cigarette lighter but doesn't smoke cigarettes; and

- she is a libertarian—and even if she's not a stoner, she won't mind if you are, so no harm in asking.

When buying cannabis from a HP, there are a few good policies to follow. First, take note: Your HP is just that—your hookup person, end of story. You don't need to know anything else about her. Unless information is offered, do not ask questions. If your friend or acquaintance offers to buy pot for you, say thank you and don't press for details or ask for introductions. It's best to treat everything on a need-to-know basis: All you need to know is when and where to go, and how much money to bring.

Granted, over time you may come to know your HP on a more personal level, and these rules might loosen. Let your HP take the lead and respond accordingly.

Here are some other points of etiquette buyers follow when dealing with HPs:

- Always bring cash, and have exact change.

- Do not haggle. This is not a South American bazaar; the price is whatever the HP says it is.

- Ignore the rule above if the HP does not deliver what was promised. If the quality is poor (and that's not what you were expecting) or the amount seems light, you have the right to politely question it. A reputable HP will then weigh it in front of you. Or you may get blown off and lose the connection altogether, but it likely wasn't worth having anyway.

- Don't ask questions that are none of your business, such as where your HP gets her weed or how much it costs her.

- Don't ask for free samples.

- Don't dawdle. Get in, do your business, get out.

- Don't bring friends unless you have arranged to do so in advance and know it is OK.

- Even if you personally know your HP, never show up unannounced unless you have prior permission to do so.

- Don't talk about the transaction on the phone, in emails, or on social media platforms. Definitely don't take photos while transacting.

- Don't draw unnecessary attention to yourself when visiting your HP. Be as low key and invisible as possible. Turn the car stereo down, and don't talk loudly on your cell phone.

- If a friend has visited a HP on your behalf to get you some marijuana, it is customary to *smoke them out*, meaning to smoke some of it together when you meet up for the exchange. It is also good stoner etiquette to give them a joint or a bud for their trouble.

- If a friend regularly procures weed for you, it's not unreasonable for her to make a little cash on the deal for her time and trouble.

SAFETY PATROL: DON'T BUY FROM COPS

This bit of advice may seem like a no-brainer, but it isn't always as easy as it sounds. Undercover cops are paid to trick you into buying from them or selling to them.

Having received a majority of their education from television police dramas, people believe a lot of myths when it comes to law enforcement. One of the most common is the assumption that an undercover police officer has to tell you he is an officer if you ask him before buying or selling drugs, soliciting for prostitution, or a host of other potentially illegal activities. Not true!

The cops are allowed to lie to you. And they will.

There is no way to definitively tell if the person you are talking to is a cop. If someone is pushing just a little too hard, it should raise a red flag. Another thing some friends and I have observed through the years is that many police officers look like your average dad type, with a gut (probably from all the paperwork), but they are in far better physical shape. Think of a fireman with a paunch. I am sure there are exceptions to this rule, but so far it's the only constant we have observed. Long hair, tattoos, piercings, scruffy appearance— none of that matters. Don't let the car fool you, either. I have seen undercovers get out of everything from beat-up old junkers to pimp mobiles to conversion vans. The best advice is to trust your woman's intuition. If something even remotely doesn't feel right, don't do it!

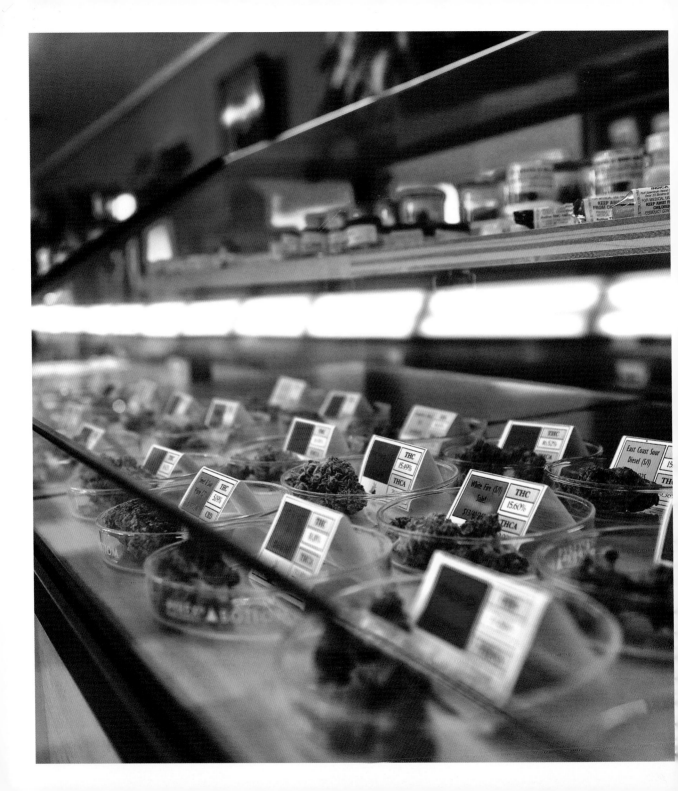

TO MARKET, TO MARKET: BUYING IN A DISPENSARY

First, let's talk about what a dispensary is: For the sake of clarity, I am going to use that term to describe shops where people—patients or otherwise—can go to purchase marijuana. They may also go by other names for legal reasons. For instance, in California you will find *collectives* and, less often, *cooperatives*. Patients become members of a nonprofit collective or cooperative. As a member they might get involved in the running of the collective and the growing of the medicine, but more often than not they will elect to simply go to the collective's dispensary to buy marijuana.

The exchange of cash for cannabis presents a bone of contention for a lot of prosecutors, who argue that medical marijuana patients must actually be involved in the cultivating of the plant for an entity to be a true collective. Luckily for a lot of seriously and terminally ill people who can barely get out of bed, let alone take up gardening, the courts in California have ruled this nonsense. But each state has different rules.

If you're lucky enough to live near a clean, well-lit dispensary, definitely check it out! Most are stocked with lots of different marijuana strains and assortments of edibles, tinctures, and concentrates. Some even sell seeds or plant clones for those who want to grow their own. If all you have dealt with is the independent market, be prepared to feel like a kid in a candy store the first time you visit a dispensary.

Can't get out to a dispensary? Use a delivery service and have the goods brought to your door. Most good services have a website or a way to send you a menu of what's in stock, so you can browse at your leisure before placing an order.

Unlike buying from a HP, it's perfectly OK to get friendly and talkative with the folks who work in a dispensary. They can help you choose the best products for your needs. Good dispensary employees LOVE to talk about marijuana and will be happy to share what they know about their stock, how it was grown, what they like and don't like, and so on. It's also a common dispensary practice to allow customers to examine (but not touch) and smell the cannabis before buying.

Just because it's a store and it's legal doesn't mean there aren't rules. If you like your dispensary and want them to stay around, be sure to follow those rules, as they are frequently under attack from uninformed reefer madness–fueled neighbors who just know in their heart of hearts that all kinds of nefarious activity is going on inside. Do your part to help your dispensary win over the community by abiding by their guidelines, which always include some variations on the following:

◀ *Dispensary inventory on display*

- Bring your ID and doctor's recommendation for verification each time you visit.

- Unless the store specifically allows it, no medicating on the premises (or on the street or in your car near the premises).

- If the dispensary does allow medicating on the premises, do so only in designated areas.

- Avoid playing loud music in your car or other activities that might disturb the neighbors.

- Don't bring friends. Only people with valid doctor's recommendations are permitted inside a medical marijuana dispensary. In states where recreational marijuana use is legal, go ahead and bring your buddies, but never bring the kids in either instance.

- In medical marijuana states, no sharing of medicine is allowed; the person who procured it must be the person to use it. Yes, people share all the time and you probably will too, but don't do it anywhere near the dispensary, where neighbors and law enforcement might be watching.

SHOPPING FOR A GOOD DISPENSARY

Some medical marijuana states take a hands-on approach to the dispensing of cannabis, passing ultra-strict rules and regulations. Others leave their laws murky and the quality of their dispensaries vary greatly depending on the integrity and acumen of their management. You might encounter some fly-by-night organizations out to make a quick buck, but don't get discouraged. Keep searching; a lot of people got into this business because they passionately believe in the power of this plant and how it can help people. Here are some things that will make a reputable dispensary stand out.

- It's brightly lit and sparkling clean.

- The employees or volunteers are friendly, helpful, and knowledgeable.

- There is security present.

- Unless there is a specific medicating area, people should not be loitering or smoking.

- The best dispensaries are in it for more than money. They offer educational programs for their members, such as growing or cooking classes, and they will also be involved in the political fight for safe legal access and encourage their members to get involved as well.

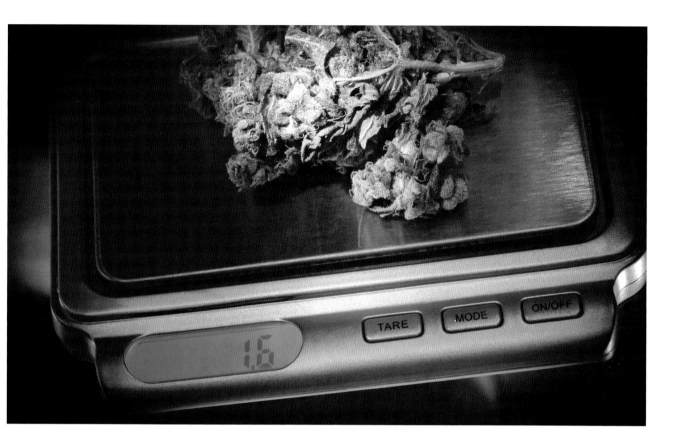

- Most importantly, a good dispensary is a place you feel comfortable and safe.

DECIPHERING A DISPENSARY MENU BOARD

A quick look at the menu board in some marijuana dispensaries might make you think you are looking at a stock chart. So many columns of numbers! What can all those prices mean?

It's simple, actually. The left-hand column will tell you the marijuana strain. The columns to the right represent the price for ascending weights: 1 gram; ⅛ ounce; ¼ ounce; ½ ounce; 1 ounce.

Depending on where you live, you may or may not be able to purchase an ounce. But legal or black market, the more you buy, the cheaper it gets. If you can afford to buy in quarter, half, or full pounds, you'll have a long-term supply at a bargain price. Of course, having that much weed could carry some serious legal consequences, even if you are a qualified patient in a medical marijuana state. As always, survey your local legal landscape and procure accordingly.

TRANSPORTING MARIJUANA

You are legally most vulnerable while driving with marijuana in the car. Needless to say, you should not smoke while driving. And even if you smoke in the car after reaching your destination, the smell can linger, so it is a good idea to avoid it (or to use some sort of odor filtration gadget—see Chapter 2). Here are some other tips to keep you and the stash you are transporting from attracting unwanted attention:

- Don't give the police a reason to stop you. Make sure all your vehicle lights are in working order and that your registration is current. Don't speed or use your cell phone.

- Keep the cannabis in your trunk so that even if you are stopped and searched, you can't be accused of driving and smoking. If you have a locked box in the trunk, so much the better.

- Fresh marijuana smells great but is a dead giveaway you have some in the car. Mitigate this by using a product designed to eliminate odor. Consider investing in Activated Carbon Fiber bags like those made by Stealth Products, which actually absorb odor. They come in a variety of sizes and styles and they really work! stealth-products.com

BUDDYING UP TO THE BUDTENDER

A good **budtender,** or the person working behind the counter at a marijuana dispensary, can be an invaluable asset. Think of budtenders as the sommeliers of marijuana. If they are knowledgeable—and in a good dispensary they will be—they can tell you all about the various strains available and their strengths and effects, which is especially helpful for newbies. A good budtender will know all about the dispensary's products and how they were grown or made. Most importantly, once they get to know you, they can make specific recommendations based on your needs and tastes, as well as alert you when particularly fine strains come in.

THE CASE OF THE DISAPPEARING DISPENSARY

Despite medical marijuana being legal in many states, law enforcement and politicians remain resistant to the idea, to the point of going against the will of the voters and working to shut down dispensaries. Sometimes local governments have even called in the federal government on their own local citizens. That's why the dispensary you visited last week might be gone this week. It's often a game of Whac-A-Mole, with one location closing, only to reopen a few blocks away to stay ahead of cities and counties that are out to ban safe access.

Because of this, many dispensaries try to keep a low profile, putting up minimal signage and doing no advertising. Vast swaths of the general public in medical marijuana states drive past them every day, oblivious to what's behind those closed doors. A green cross is the most common giveaway that you've happened upon a dispensary. Also look for buzzwords like "Compassionate Care," "Alternative Healing," and "Herbal Healing."

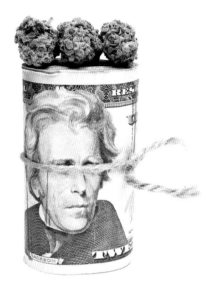

WHY IS A WEED SO EXPENSIVE?

Americans spend huge amounts of money trying to get rid of weeds every year, so why is this particular weed so expensive, costing hundreds of dollars an ounce?

In a word, risk.

Sure, there are expenses involved with growing marijuana, especially indoor hydroponic marijuana (see Chapter 8 for details), but not enough to merit the prices charged by dealers and dispensaries alike.

If you live in a state that criminalizes marijuana, the person transporting and selling marijuana is taking an enormous risk, including felony charges and substantial prison time. Any time there is that much risk involved, people need to be compensated for it.

Even in states where marijuana is legal or quasilegal, it remains illegal at the federal level, so some risk is always involved. Whatever protections state law provides are more than made up for in taxes and fees, which add to the expense. Those often exceed what any other business has to pay, for in their misguided efforts to curb marijuana use, officials often try to make it cost-prohibitive. What this actually accomplishes is to put further financial hardship on sick patients who really need cannabis as medicine, and it drives both medical and recreational users back to the black market.

"It's ridiculous that we continue to incarcerate anyone for using a substance that actually causes far less damage than alcohol. . . . No one should be jailed for possessing marijuana."

—*Susan Sarandon*

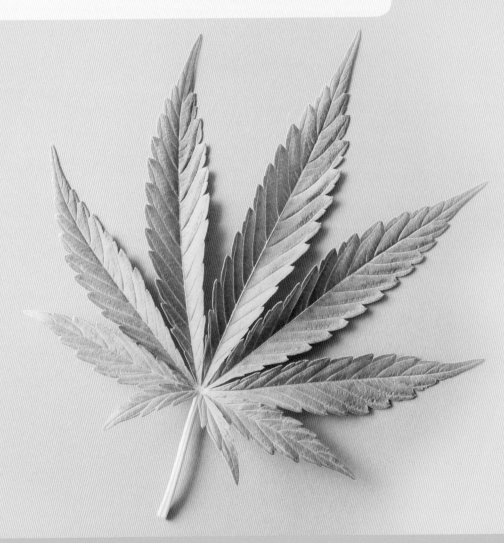

CHAPTER 5

WEED *the* PEOPLE: KNOW YOUR RIGHTS

The number-one rule when it comes to avoiding legal snafus is Don't Break the Law.

That's the truth, and you should remember it, though it's not as simple as it sounds. Cannabis law is complicated. And here's the sad reality when it comes to marijuana: With few exceptions, the police are not your friends. It's vitally important for all cannabis users, even those in legal or medicinally legal states, to know their rights. This means knowing what to do and say and, more importantly, what NOT to do and say, if you happen to have an encounter with law enforcement.

I'm not a lawyer, but there are some conventional wisdoms I can share with you. The vast majority of casual cannabis users won't ever have a problem with the police, but some will. Lest you think it can never happen to you, more than 750,000 people were arrested for marijuana-related offenses in the United States in 2011 (the last year for which data are available), 87 percent of them for mere possession. Learn the material in this chapter, just in case.

Oaksterdam University in Oakland, California, the industry's leading educational center for those seeking careers in cannabis, stresses to its students over and over again to always think in terms of risk management. The professors preach that, whenever you are dealing with marijuana, you should act in such a way that, if the worst ever happens, you have given your attorney the tools she needs to successfully defend you. In a nutshell, that means you need to understand your rights under the law and not get tricked into giving those rights away.

That's good advice for casual users as well. Even if an arrest for possession doesn't yield you jail time, it can still turn into an expensive, time-consuming hassle. It can also cause serious consequences like suspension of your driver's license, mandatory drug rehab programs, loss of student funding, loss of public housing and other public assistance, and diminished job opportunities. Prison time is never completely out of the question either, especially if you have prior convictions, as did the Louisiana man who got twenty years for possessing about a half ounce of marijuana.

Never expect the police to be on your side. Their ultimate goal—to make an arrest that will result in a criminal conviction—is in direct conflict with your goal to stay out of trouble with the law. Lying is part of their job. I have personally heard police officers proudly testify to this fact in court.

Be aware:

- The police do not have to read you your rights unless they intend to question you about a specific crime, and then only after you are arrested. A lot of people mistakenly think their case must be dismissed if they weren't read their rights. Not true! That may affect the admissibility of what you say, but it won't make your case disappear.

- The police do not have to let you know you have the right to refuse a search, and they are allowed to try to intimidate you into agreeing to one. Most searches happen not because the police have the legally required probable cause, but

because people got tricked into giving consent. If an officer has to ask you if he can search your person, car, or home, he probably doesn't have probable cause. ALWAYS refuse to consent to searches.

- Don't be fooled into talking or otherwise "cooperating" by the promise that things will go easier for you if you do. That is a lie. Anything you say at any time can and will be used against you. Be sure your friends and family understand this fact because if you get arrested with others, the police will separate you and try to play you against each other, including lying about what your friend supposedly told them.

THE CONSTITUTION HAS YOUR BACK . . . IF YOU LET IT

You may not win any friends on the force by asserting your rights, but, if the cops realize that you know your rights, they might be more cautious about violating those rights. By invoking any of the three lines in the sidebar, you have protection under the Bill of Rights of the US Constitution. Vary from those lines and start chatting with the police and that protection vanishes like a puff of smoke. Let's explore why.

SAFETY PATROL:

No Chatting

Any police encounter can induce a lot of stress. The police know this and will use it to their advantage to get you to talk. Anything you say, even in casual conversation, can be used against you. No matter how innocent and friendly they act, DO NOT CHAT WITH THE POLICE. No matter how threatening and intimidating they can be, DO NOT CHAT WITH THE POLICE. They will find ways to trip you up. Remember what I said about giving your attorney the best tools to defend you if the worst should ever happen? Listen up and shut up! These are the only things you should ever say during an encounter with the police in regard to your marijuana use (and probably at any other time too):

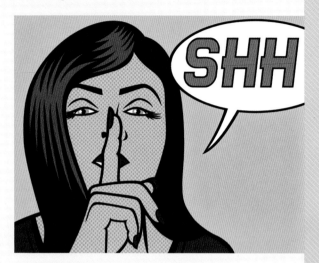

- "I do not consent to a search."

- "Officer, are you detaining me, or am I free to go?"

- "I choose to remain silent until I can speak to an attorney."

That's it. No more! Ingrain those three lines into your brain, and, if law enforcement ever stops you, stick by them. Practice scenarios with your friends so that everyone is prepared for a law enforcement encounter, in case it ever happens. In the heat of the moment, even people who know better get flustered and forget. Do not flinch. Only these three lines!

"I do not consent to a search."

In order for the police to search you, they either need a search warrant signed by a judge or "probable cause." That means the officer must have seen something tangible, such as drugs or paraphernalia, in order to believe a crime is taking place. Anything in plain sight is fair game, so if an officer looks through the windows of the car or peeps in the door to your house and sees anything potentially illegal, he or she has the right to come in and search.

Don't worry about whether the officer has or says he has probable cause to search you, your vehicle, or your home because you always have the right to refuse searches. In and of itself, refusing a search is not an admission of any kind of guilt and it does not give the officer the right to search or detain you.

Sometimes the police will search anyway, but saying "no" is about more than stopping the search from taking place. It's about arming your potential defense attorney with the tools to defend you. If the police search without your consent, your attorney can challenge the search. If the judge agrees the police did not have probable cause to execute a search, the search and any evidence it gathered will be thrown out, and likely your entire case along with it.

"But what if I have nothing to hide?"

Many people think if they have done nothing wrong and have nothing to hide, it won't hurt to let the police search. Keep the cops happy, and get it over with so they'll move on.

Refer again to the list of the only things you should say during a law enforcement encounter. Ever. Period. NEVER CONSENT TO A SEARCH!

Why not?

- At best, searches are messy. The police will tear through your belongings, house, and/or car like a tornado, leaving a huge mess in their wake.

- Things may get damaged, including expensive things like computers and televisions. If you consented to the search, you may not be entitled to collect damages, and, even if you are, actually collecting on said damages can be a time-consuming, frustrating, bureaucratic nightmare of red tape.

- I am not accusing the cops of stealing but . . . valuable personal items like jewelry and cash mysteriously disappear during searches all the time.

- You never know what has been left in your car by someone who borrowed it, or what a friend dropped at your house, or what is in the pocket of the clothes you're wearing. Any evidence found, even something as small as a roach, will be used against you if you consented to a search, whether you knew about it or not.

- I am by no means saying that all police are this corrupt, but evidence planting happens. Never consent to a search.

"Officer, are you detaining me, or am I free to go?"

A lot of people fail to realize that, unless you are actually being formally detained, taken into custody, or arrested, you have the right to terminate a law enforcement encounter at any time by simply asking the officer if you are free to go. The officer may keep pressing you to talk or further try to intimidate you into giving up your rights, but she does not have the right to keep you unless she is prepared to formally detain you. In that case, she has to have some sort of "reasonable suspicion" that you have committed a crime.

Clearly asking if you are free to go can help your lawyer, should you ever go to court, because it demonstrates the encounter was not voluntary. If the officer is not prepared to arrest you, she has to let you go.

Practice that line a few times and get comfortable with it. Do not wait to be dismissed. Exercise your rights and say, "Officer, are you detaining me, or am I free to go?"

"I choose to remain silent until I can speak to an attorney."

Everyone has the right to remain silent when dealing with the police, and everyone accused of a crime in the United States has the right to legal representation by an attorney. If you can't afford an attorney, one will be appointed for you.

The only time you should talk to the police is in the physical presence of your attorney. This third line will only come into play if the first two didn't work and you find yourself being formally detained. Stay calm, and, aside from that one line, keep your

mouth shut until your lawyer can advise you. Yes, the Supreme Court ruled that you do actually need to verbally assert your right to remain silent and request an attorney, but that's it. No more talking until you see your lawyer.

According to Los Angeles defense attorney Michael Levinsohn, the standard Miranda warning is incomplete anyway. Here's how Levinsohn says the warning should read for a better real life explanation of what Miranda means:

You have the right to remain silent. Anything you say can be used against you. Whatever you say cannot be introduced by you or your attorney in your defense, since that is inadmissible hearsay. Only the prosecution can use it, and then only against you. However, your decision to remain silent cannot be used against you. You have the right to an attorney, but, if you cannot afford one, you will only get one when you are brought to court in a couple of days. Likewise, even if you can afford one, it will be several hours, long after the police are finished with you and you have been booked into a jail somewhere before you will actually see that attorney.

Don't Get Fooled by Drug Checkpoint Traps

Listen up, my little buds—this is important! Even though the Supreme Court has ruled that random checkpoints set up for the purpose of finding illegal drugs are unconstitutional, the police know that most citizens don't know this.

So they sometimes put up signs on the highway warning of an upcoming drug checkpoint ahead. They know they can't legally search cars for no reason, but they are looking for people who make illegal U-turns, pull off into the next rest area, get off at the next exit, or otherwise try to evade the checkpoint. If you ever see such a sign and you have marijuana in the car, take a deep breath, stay calm, and just keep driving. Most of the time, there is no such checkpoint ahead and that's the end of it. The folks who try to evade the phony checkpoint, however, will likely have their vehicles examined by drug-sniffing dogs.

Keep in mind that officers may not keep you at roadside waiting for a dog to arrive for no reason. They can only take as much time as is necessary to complete the tasks of citing you for any traffic violations committed in your haste to avoid the checkpoint.

Some law enforcement agencies have been known to push the legal envelope with the drug checkpoint tactic. Just because the police act like they have the right to randomly search cars does not mean they actually do. If you do get stopped in an alleged random drug checkpoint, treat it like any other traffic stop and limit your conversation to the three lines you should say during a law enforcement encounter, starting with (repeat after me, ladies):

"I do not consent to a search."

WHAT TO DO IF YOU ARE STOPPED BY THE POLICE ON THE STREET

You are not necessarily required to show your ID on request for no reason, although this differs from state to state. Check your local laws by calling the local office of the American Civil Liberties Union.

Do not consent to a search. If the officer suspects you have a weapon, he has the right to pat you down, but he may NOT reach into your pockets unless he sees something immediately recognizable as a weapon or contraband. Never chat. Simply assert your rights, remain silent, and politely inquire if you are free to leave. If you are detained, assert your right to remain silent until you can speak to an attorney.

WHAT TO DO IF YOU ARE STOPPED BY THE POLICE IN YOUR CAR

Traffic stops make up roughly 50 percent of citizen police encounters. The same rules apply: Do not chat. Especially, do not admit to doing anything wrong, even if you did. For instance, saying, "I'm sorry, officer, I know I was speeding." BAD IDEA. You just admitted to a crime.

Stay in your car with your hands in view until the officer approaches. Open the window only enough to communicate and hand out your license and registration, which you are required to show when operating a vehicle. This makes it more difficult for the officer to poke his head inside and look into or smell inside the car. Remember, anything he sees in plain sight is fair game, and the scent of cannabis (real or imagined) constitutes enough probable cause to search your car.

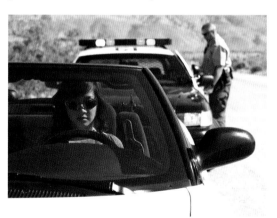

Airport security personnel do not need probable cause or a warrant to search you or your belongings. Neither do border guards and immigration officers any time you enter or leave a country.

Security also has the right to search your person and belongings as a condition of entering certain locations and private events such as courthouses and other federal facilities, sporting events, concerts, nightclubs, amusement parks, and festivals. More often than not, weapons are the targets of these searches, but it's best not to chance it. If private security officers find anything illegal, they can turn it over to the police.

If you are attending a private event at which search is a condition of entry, the required search MUST take place upon entering. If they ask to search you afterward, you have the right to refuse and to leave without submitting to the search.

If you and your passengers are asked to get out of the car, do so and close and lock the doors behind you. Yes, even if you end up locking your keys in the car. Oops, just chalk it up to habit. Whether or not you retain your keys, closing and locking the door makes it more difficult for the police to search, and they will have to be really determined and get a warrant to do so.

Again, verbally assert your right to remain silent and politely inquire if you are free to leave.

Time is on your side during a traffic stop. If the encounter takes long enough, the officers will get a call to attend to something more important than looking for a little reefer in your Road Warrior. They'll have to leave

and you'll be free to go. The same can happen during street encounters.

WHAT TO DO IF THE POLICE COME TO YOUR HOME

Of all the places police can search, your home enjoys the most protection under the law.

According to Levinsohn, a search of a house or structure always requires a warrant, unless the police perceive an emergency or believe someone's life is in danger.

There's only one rule when dealing with the police at home, and it's a simple one. Never allow the police into your home unless they have a warrant. Period.

If the police come to your door, open the door as little as possible, step outside, close the door behind you, and talk to them outside. If they ask if they can come in or look around, there is one line you can safely say, besides the three outlined in the sidebar:

"Do you have a warrant? I'm sorry, officer, I can't let you in without a warrant."

From there, assert your right to refuse any kind of search, even if they threaten to come back with a warrant.

SHOCKING!

How Marijuana Became Federally Illegal

It all happened so quickly the public barely had time to notice. Congress held only two short hearings, lasting under one hour, to debate the merits of marijuana prohibition.

Prior to 1937, Harry Anslinger, head of the newly formed Bureau of Narcotics—essentially the nation's first drug czar—with help from William Randolph Hearst and other industrial magnates who all stood to significantly increase their fortunes in paper, oil, and other commodities if hemp were made illegal, had been lobbying hard against "marihuana."

Most Americans had no idea that this strange foreign word that Hearst's newspapers regularly blamed for all manner of violence, insanity, and death—told in lurid, racist, yellow journalism—was the same cannabis they had in their medicine cabinets at home.

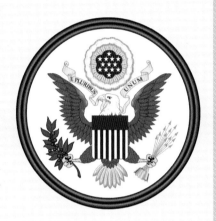

A little thing called the Constitution prevented the government from just outlawing marijuana, but Anslinger found a way around that by introducing legislation that made taxes on cannabis cost-prohibitive and levied fines and prison time on anyone not obeying them.

When it came time for Congress to decide, Anslinger testified before the House Ways and Means Committee about how the drug is "entirely the monster-Hyde, the harmful effect of which cannot be measured." Treasury Department Assistant General Counsel Clinton Hester backed up Anslinger's claims, stating that marijuana's eventual effect was "death."

That was enough for the committee. No facts, no science, just the ridiculous rantings of a powerful man with an agenda. The entirety of the hearings took an hour before the committee approved the *Marijuana Stamp Tax Act*. The House of Representatives gave the matter less debate, passing the bill in a mere 90 seconds, with only two questions posed. First, Speaker of the House Sam Rayburn was asked to summarize the bill. His concise answer: "I don't know. It has something to do with a thing called marijuana. I think it is a narcotic of some kind."

Rayburn was then asked whether or not the American Medical Association supported the bill. A member of the committee falsely reported that the association had given the measure its full support, when in fact the AMA represented the lone voice against marijuana prohibition before Congress in 1937. With that brief exchange, federal marijuana prohibition in the United States began. The heavy-handed enforcement of the nation's drug laws in the years ahead had to go beyond any of Harry Anslinger's wildest dreams. After all, he believed alcohol prohibition would have worked, if only the punishments had been harsher.

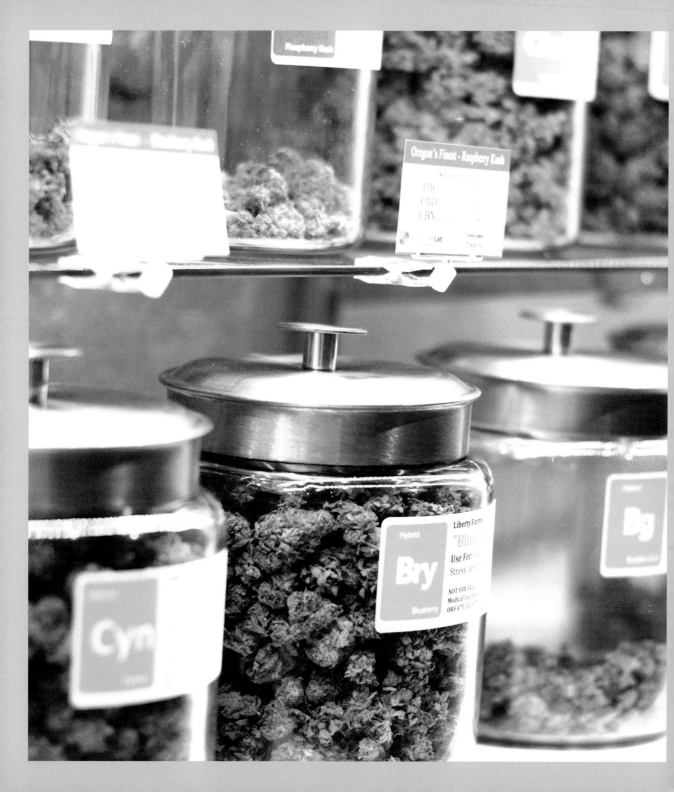

CHAPTER 6

PAGING DR. MARY JANE: MEDICAL MARIJUANA

Prohibitionists like to laugh at the idea of marijuana as medicine. They say it doesn't make sense: How can a single plant treat ailments as disparate as wasting syndrome and obesity, autism and alcoholism, psoriasis and brain tumors?

The joke is on them. This single plant can treat all those conditions and hundreds more. It may sound unbelievable, but, like many things associated with marijuana, the facts run counterintuitive to what seems logical. Once you understand the science about how cannabis works in the body, it makes perfect sense.

Exciting things are happening in the world of cannabis medicine. New research emerges every day that shows its promise in treating a wide range of illnesses and ailments, from minor to terminal. One of

◀ *Glass storage jars keep dispensary inventory in perfect cured condition*

the biggest overall changes we are seeing—compared to the research done prior to the 1990s—is the exploration of the ability of cannabis to not only treat symptoms of diseases but to actually cure the afflictions themselves. Cannabis has been shown to be effective in treating such diverse conditions as:

- ALS (Lou Gehrig's disease)
- Alzheimer's disease
- Autism
- Bipolar disorder
- Cardiovascular disease
- Crohn's disease
- A variety of other gastrointestinal disorders
- Depression

- Epilepsy

- Hepatitis C

- HIV

- Lupus

- A variety of other autoimmune conditions

- PTSD (Post-traumatic stress disorder)

- Multiple sclerosis

- Stroke

The list of afflictions that have not been treated by cannabis would be far shorter than those that have! Let's explore some of the most common cannabis uses for women and how they might help you or someone you love.

THE BIG C

Unlike a lot of overly enthusiastic cannabis advocates, you won't hear me making the blanket statement, "Cannabis cures cancer." What kind of cancer? At what stage? In whom? How and how much? With or without what other therapies? Let's face it, the word encompasses a whole lot of very different diseases.

That said, many credible studies on cannabis and cancer do show that a potential cure might be found in this plant. Unlike chemotherapy, which kills everything, cannabis has

> " The science is there. This isn't ancedotal. "
>
> —*Dr. Sanjay Gupta*

demonstrated the ability to selectively target cancer cells while leaving healthy cells intact.

As of this writing, I am comfortable saying that cannabis can cure some cancers, some of the time. I long for the day when the government allows us to learn how to use it to its full potential so we will be able to talk about cancer and cannabis without any qualifiers or reservations. Nonetheless, right now we do know that cannabis fights cancer in a number of ways. It is

- antiproliferative—it stops cancer cells from reproducing;

- anti-angiogenic—it prevents the formation of blood vessels that are necessary for cancerous tumors to grow;

- antimetastatic—it prevents cancer from spreading to other organs; and

- apoptotic—it induces cancer cells to destroy themselves.

A 2009 study conducted by a team of researchers from several leading universities and published in the journal *Cancer Prevention Research* found that long-term,

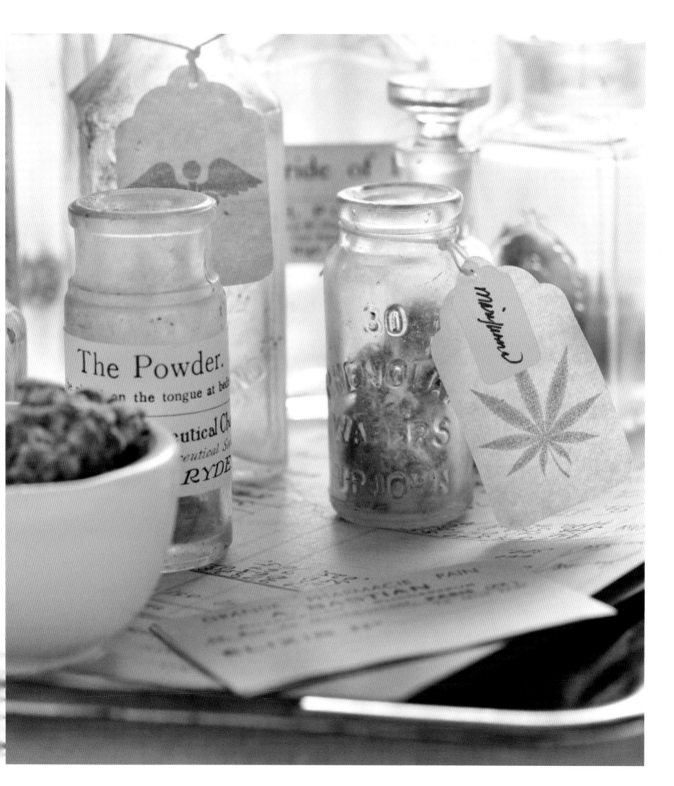

moderate marijuana smokers have *significantly* (48 percent) lower incidences of squamous cell cancers of the head and neck than those who abstain. Medical research from around the globe, in laboratory, animal, and/or human studies and trials, also shows positive results in treating gliomas (brain tumors), lymphomas, and cancers of the breast, prostate, lung, uterus, cervix, mouth, colon, biliary tract, thyroid, pancreas, and skin.

DIABETES

Researchers believe marijuana can help regulate your metabolism and control inflammation, which play crucial roles in diabetes pathology. Scientists are still not sure exactly why, but a study published in the *American Journal of Epidemiology* showed that despite marijuana's ability to increase appetite (aka "the munchies"), overall obesity rates for cannabis users weighed in at about a third less than their abstaining counterparts, even when taking external factors into account. If marijuana somehow helps regulate metabolism and weight, we shouldn't be surprised to learn it also holds promise in treating Type II diabetes, a disease that affects more than 300 million people worldwide.

FEMALE TROUBLE

Cannabis was used in obstetrics and gynecology long before there were such things as gynecologists and obstetricians. Mary Jane can, in fact, help women through the stages of reproductive life. Forgo pain meds and try it the next time you are particularly bothered by painful menstrual cramps, or to ease the mood swings and hot flashes of menopause, as women have for thousands of years.

Besides its cancer-fighting potential, cannabis therapy has shown promise in treating some serious afflictions that primarily affect women, although in all cases more research is needed to understand exactly how and why it works. What we do know is:

- Women make up 80–90 percent of *fibromyalgia* patients, according to the National Institutes of Health. A painful condition characterized by chronic musculoskeletal pain, the disorder manifests many symptoms that respond to cannabis therapy, including chronic pain, joint stiffness, and sleep disturbances. Sometimes these symptoms lead to anxiety and depression, also helped by Mary Jane.

- A degenerative bone disease characterized by deteriorating bone tissue, **osteoporosis** puts patients at greater risk of serious multiple bone fractures. Worldwide, one in three women over age fifty will experience fractures related to osteoporosis (as will one in five men). While the exact role the endocannabinoid system plays in regulating bone mass is not yet understood, preclinical research shows promise in reducing bone loss, stimulating bone formation, and slowing the progression of the disease.

- *Rheumatoid arthritis,* an autoimmune disease characterized by chronic inflammatory polyarthritis (arthritis that affects five or more joints), is more prevalent in women, although it affects only about 1 percent of the population. Along with a lot of anecdotal evidence conducted by surveys of cannabis-using patients, preclinical research shows promise in slowing the disease's progression, especially when cannabidiol is used. Furthermore, researchers at the British Royal National Hospital for Rheumatic Disease found that cannabis extracts, administered over a five-week period, demonstrated significant improvements over placebos in relieving pain while moving and resting, decreasing pain intensity and inflammation, and improving sleep quality.

- According to the American Thyroid Association, women are five to eight times more likely than men to have *thyroid* problems. One woman in eight will develop a thyroid disorder during her lifetime. Scientists don't know exactly how cannabis affects the over- or underactive thyroid gland, but we do know that endocannabinoid receptors are abundant both in the thyroid gland and in the parts of the brain that send signals to that gland. Regardless of how it works, patients report that cannabis helps with the symptoms attached to the disorders, providing relief from pain, insomnia, anxiety, depression, and more.

MATERNITY AND MARIJUANA

Pregnancy is another one of those hot button topics that makes uninformed people's heads explode. But even disregarding the thousands of years of historical evidence of women successfully using cannabis to treat nausea, labor pains, and other afflictions associated with pregnancy and childbirth, the safety of marijuana overall has been tested far more than the prescription drugs typically given to pregnant women to treat morning sickness and some of its more severe side effects.

Both mother and fetus have endocannabinoid systems and naturally occurring endocannabinoids, and we already know that you cannot overdose on cannabis. But does it adversely affect the developing fetus? Unfortunately, it is almost impossible for doctors and researchers to get permission to conduct any kind of study that exposes unborn children to marijuana, and the few studies we have from the U.S. government fail to take into account the mother's use of other drugs and alcohol.

Furthermore, pregnant women who admit to using cannabis can face serious consequences, especially if they live in prohibitionist states like Texas or Oklahoma, although nobody is completely safe, even in medical marijuana states. As long as women have reason to fear legal prosecution for child endangerment or child abuse as a result of using medical cannabis, it will be impossible to get a true reading of how many of them are already doing so and the outcomes of their experiences. Once again, politics stands directly in the way of medical progress.

The credible research we do have shows potential benefits to both mothers, especially those suffering from extreme nausea and vomiting that can endanger the life of their unborn child, and their children. Several

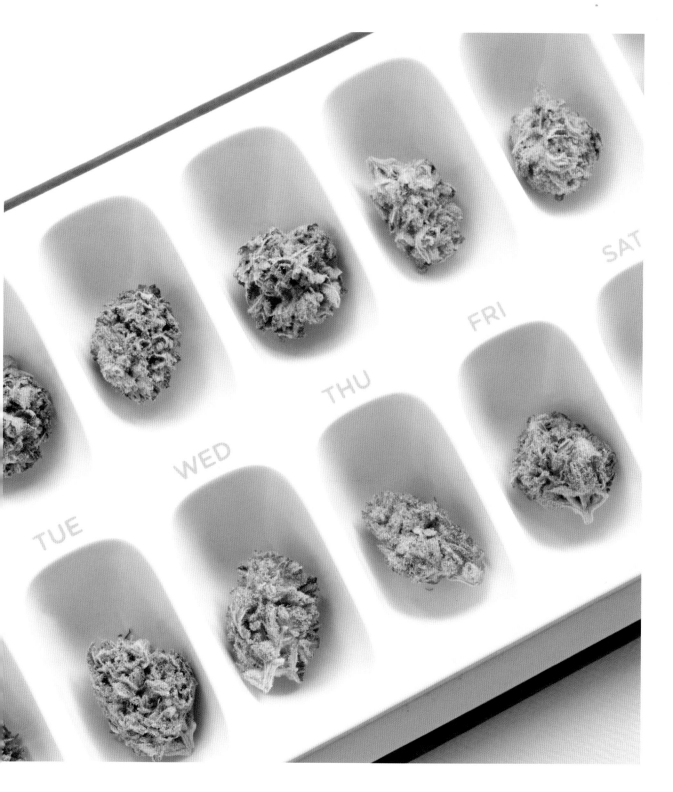

MEET THC'S LESSER KNOWN COUSIN, CBD

While scientists are just beginning to research the over sixty cannabinoids and what they do, one cannabinoid is beginning to stand out. Unlike THC, it will not get you high but shows great promise in treating a variety of ailments.

Cannabidiol, or *CBD*, has analgesic, antispasmodic, anxiolytic, antipsychotic, anti-emetic, antibacterial, and anti-inflammatory properties. Clinical studies show CBD to have neuroprotective properties as well: It shows promise in treating stroke, brain injuries, and alcohol-induced toxicity. Studies have also shown CBD to possess anti-tumor properties by inhibiting tumor growth while inducing apoptosis in malignant cells. CBD counts are typically higher in indica strains—this is the component that gives marijuana its sedative effect.

Because of CBD's outstanding medicinal properties, growers and breeders are now beginning to look beyond the high of THC and cultivate strains specifically for their non-psychoactive high CBD content.

studies show that cannabis use by the mother does not affect birth weight or gestation periods. Most compelling is Dr. Melanie Dreher's study of marijuana-using Jamaican mothers, published in 1994. One of the largest studies on neonatal outcomes among mothers using cannabis during pregnancy and breastfeeding, it not only examined the infants at birth but also tracked them through early development, testing to compare their progress against babies not exposed to cannabis.

The researchers chose Jamaica for the study because of the country's cultural acceptance of marijuana use over a wide range of socioeconomic groups, and because use of other drugs and even alcohol among the test subjects was low.

Dreher's study found no significant physical or psychological differences at three days old between the babies of mothers who were heavy cannabis users and babies of mothers who did not use cannabis. At one month old, the children whose mothers used marijuana performed better on a variety of physiological and autonomic tests than the nonexposed children, although this latter trend may have resulted from socioeconomic factors.

MORE MARY JANE FOR
WHAT AILS YOU

When you listen to politicians debate the merits of legalizing medical marijuana, they almost always talk about serious, devastating, sometimes fatal, diseases like cancer. But even minor ailments can benefit from cannabis therapy. You might just save yourself a trip to the drugstore for all kinds of over-the-counter meds by toking up instead!

- The analgesic properties of cannabis help ease all kinds of minor (and even major) *aches and pains.* The exact mechanisms still need study, but in 2013 a team of Chinese researchers published findings that showed an important link between cannabis and acupuncture, also used to treat pain, when they found that electro acupuncture—an electrified version of traditional treatment—works by stimulating cannabinoid receptors.

- Patients report relief from cannabis from everything from minor *tension headaches* to *migraines.* In the former it is likely the ability of cannabis to help people relax and ease stress. In the latter it's believed the marijuana helps control vascular spasms that might be one of the root causes of the migraine. It can also treat symptoms like nausea and vomiting that often accompany the severe headaches.

- If you have trouble falling asleep or the quality of your sleep is lacking, a nice mellow indica strain, preferably taken in an edible form about an hour or so before bedtime, will usually help *insomnia.*

- Hundreds of peer-reviewed articles tout the benefits of marijuana for *nausea* and *vomiting,* often as a result of serious disease, but it also works for everyday minor occurrences.

- Marijuana can ease the symptoms of both chronic and occasional *gastrointestinal disorders,* including *cramping, pain,* and *inflammation.*

- About 18,000 Americans die each year from *Methicillin-resistant Staphylococcus aureus (MRSA),* and about 100,000 more are made ill by these serious antibiotic-resistant bacterial infections. British and Italian researchers reported in the *Journal of Natural Products* that THC and four other cannabis compounds showed powerful antibacterial activity against six different strains of MRSA.

- Cannabis has been shown to relieve the tics suffered by some *Tourette's syndrome* patients.

DID YOU KNOW?

Cannabis pollen found on the mummy of **Ramesses II** (d. 1213 BC) in Egypt provides evidence of the earliest recorded use there. The Egyptians used marijuana to treat diseases of the eye, presumably glaucoma; to reduce inflammatory ailments; and for "women's conditions," including the pain of childbirth.

The **Victorians** used marijuana, on its own and incorporated into a variety of proprietary medicines, for an array of maladies such as rheumatism, convulsions, muscle spasms, epilepsy, and rabies. Victorian women took cannabis in the form of an alcohol-based tincture to promote uterine contractions in childbirth or to find relief from menstrual cramps.

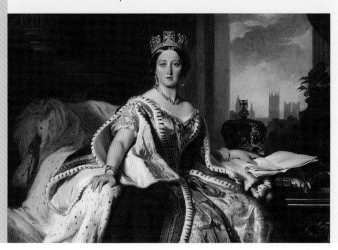

While it's been widely reported that **Queen Victoria** herself used cannabis tincture to treat her own painful menstrual cramps, we have no actual proof of this. However, the story is likely true because Sir Robert Russell, the queen's personal physician, wrote extensively about using cannabis for this purpose.

The world's oldest known complete medical textbook, the *Ebers Papyrus*, contains directions for mixing **cannabis and honey** to be introduced into the vagina to reduce inflammation in the uterus!

- While it may sound counterintuitive that something smoked could actually help a lung condition, the fact is that marijuana is a bronchial dilator, meaning it helps open airways and can be effective for *asthma, emphysema,* and other *bronchial conditions.*

- People suffering from *Lyme disease,* a bacterial inflammatory condition, especially the chronic variety, suffer from extreme pain. Cannabis has been shown to relive both the pain and inflammation caused by this debilitating condition that begins with a bite from an infected tick.

- As much as prohibitionists like to paint marijuana as a gateway drug, research shows it holds great promise as an exit drug from *alcohol and drug dependence,* by helping reduce cravings for alcohol and other addictive drugs.

- While cannabis is known to improve overall sleep quality and treat insomnia, one preclinical study on rats suggests it could play a role in reducing incidents of *sleep apnea*, a condition characterized by interrupted breathing of 10 seconds or more, that is associated with a host of other serious afflictions, including heart attack and stroke.

MARIJUANA FOR FLUFFY AND FIDO

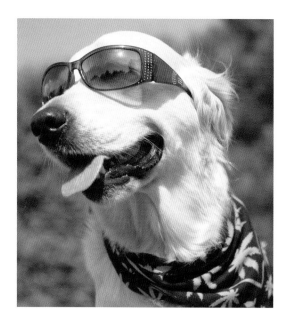

Every six months or so, you'll see some big story in the media about a new "epidemic" of people seeking veterinary care because their pets accidently ate their herb or medicated edibles. Some news stories have even inaccurately reported that marijuana is toxic to pets. Not true. Think about it: Fluffy and Fido have natural endocannabinoid systems just as we do. In fact, every animal higher on the evolutionary chain than a mollusk does. So, like people, pets are not going to overdose and die solely from ingesting cannabis. That said, animals, especially small ones, will need far less marijuana to affect them. They can certainly ingest too much, stumble around, be disoriented, and so on, like a human who has ingested too much. It may also take them longer to sleep off the effects.

I am not advocating that you feed your pet medicated edibles, but I am saying that it's not the cannabis that is risky. However, common foods such as chocolate that are frequently used in making edibles can be toxic to pets.

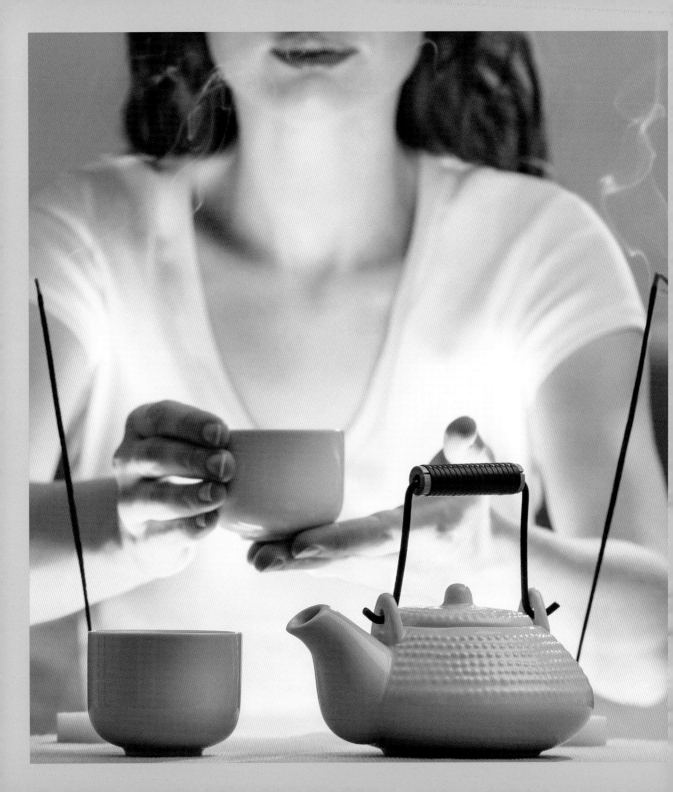

CHAPTER 7

YOGANJA!
HEALTHY LIVING *with* MARY JANE

We're all familiar with the lifestyle choices that can support healthy living and prevent our bodies from breaking down: a balanced diet, regular exercise, and enough rest, water, vitamins, and minerals. If things get really bad, in some cases, the body can be repaired with surgery.

According to Dr. Robert Melamede, one of the field's leading researchers, because of the ravages of modern living—poor diet, the prevalence of toxic chemicals, lack of exercise, and so on—most people are now endocannabinoid-deficient. That means our bodies' natural endocannabinoids, which help to maintain homeostasis, just can't keep up with everything they need to do in order to maintain optimum health. Hence the need for supplemental cannabis, which binds with the endocannabinoid receptors already inside us. Together with your natural endocannabinoids, the supplemental cannabinoids—taken in the form of marijuana—can give the body more ammunition to fight disease and the effects of aging.

Ingesting marijuana can be one of the most important preventative health practices for your anti-breakdown routine. At the biological level, the ravages of aging can be attributed to the effects of free radicals and out-of-control inflammation, both of which can be combated by the strong antioxidant properties of marijuana and a smoothly functioning endocannabinoid system.

In other words . . . yes, ladies, Mary Jane is good for you! It's good for your body, your skin, your sleep, and your overall endurance. It might even help to keep you trim! It's a powerful and potent elixir that's gentle on the system and beneficial in all kinds of surprising and exciting ways.

MARIJUANA AND EXERCISE: TWO GREAT THINGS THAT GO GREAT TOGETHER

Health professionals never cease to point out the importance of a regular exercise routine to maintain optimum health, as well as a toned physique. These same professionals usually fall short of recognizing the connection between cannabis and working out, but the truth is the proverbial runner's high has a lot in common with the marijuana high.

My personal introduction to the joy—not to mention the increased results—of working out high came from a famous plastic surgeon acquaintance who prefers to remain anonymous. This physician, himself a workout fanatic, always included smoking marijuana in his pre-run warm-up routine. Taking his advice, I started trying it before heading to the gym, an activity that usually bored me. To my surprise, the time went far faster and I was better able to concentrate on my workout rather than on how much I disliked it.

As much as I enjoy the mental stimulation offered by working out on cannabis, there are important physical benefits as well. Studies show that exercise increases endocannabinoid activity, meaning you might feel that "runner's high," which inspires so many people to keep exercising, a little easier and a little sooner. Counterintuitive as it may sound, even in its smoked form cannabis causes bronchial and vasodilation, delivering increased oxygen to the body. Marijuana's analgesic, anti-inflammatory, and antispasmodic properties can even help with the aches and pains associated with physical activity.

WEED IMPROVES EXERCISE . . . AND VICE VERSA!

It's easy to see how marijuana can improve the quality of your workout, but can your workout improve the quality of your weed? The answer appears to be yes! A 2013 University of Sydney study published in the journal *Drug and Alcohol Dependence* reported that marijuana users' THC levels increased by 15 percent after they did cardiovascular exercise, meaning that exercise might even help your inferior weed feel more potent.

CANNABIS CAN HELP TO MAINTAIN A HEALTHY BODY WEIGHT

While cannabis gets a bad rap (and a fair share of jokes on Comedy Central) for bringing on "the munchies," or an increase in hunger, that doesn't necessarily mean that marijuana is going to pack on the pounds.

Science is just beginning to explore the reasons that, as a group, marijuana users have lower body mass indexes and lower rates of diabetes than the general U.S. population. Studies show this to be the case, despite marijuana's famous ability to stimulate the appetite and cause the munchies.

That means that Mary Jane can actually help you maintain a more svelte physique! Here's how you can make weed work for you and your healthy-weight goals:

- Use the heightened sensory perception of being high to your advantage. Pick a healthy food you don't normally consider that exciting—say celery, or rice cakes, or yogurt—and eat it slowly. Appreciate all its unique properties you might have missed in the past. What does it look like? What went into creating it so you could enjoy it? Notice the texture, and revel in the crisp crunch or creamy smoothness. Notice its flavor nuances, its aroma, and more.

- Don't let boredom sabotage your diet. If you're hungry and you invite Mary Jane to dinner, chances are you'll discover some new favorite foods. Marijuana has a way of making everything taste better, so let it open the door to new healthy gastronomic experiences. When eating out, try a new ethnic cuisine, or perhaps a vegan restaurant, or eat from the vegetarian menu for some or all of your meals. When shopping, pick out a vegetable you've never tried or even heard of before and learn how to prepare it. Search for healthy recipes in magazines or online.

- Take a moment to visualize how the healthy foods you are eating will help you achieve your healthy body goals by giving your body the nutrients it needs without the excess fat, calories, or chemicals it doesn't need.

420 YOGA POSES

A growing number of yoga studios, in legal and medicinally legal states, are openly embracing the cannabis-exercise connection by offering 420-friendly classes that encourage students to participate "under the influence."

When you think about it, the concept isn't so revolutionary. Considering marijuana's use in ancient cultures, it is very possible that ancient yogis used ganja to enhance their practice.

Physically, marijuana can help relax the body, helping practitioners go deeper into asanas, or yoga poses. But most people cite more cerebral reasons for taking Mary Jane along to yoga class.

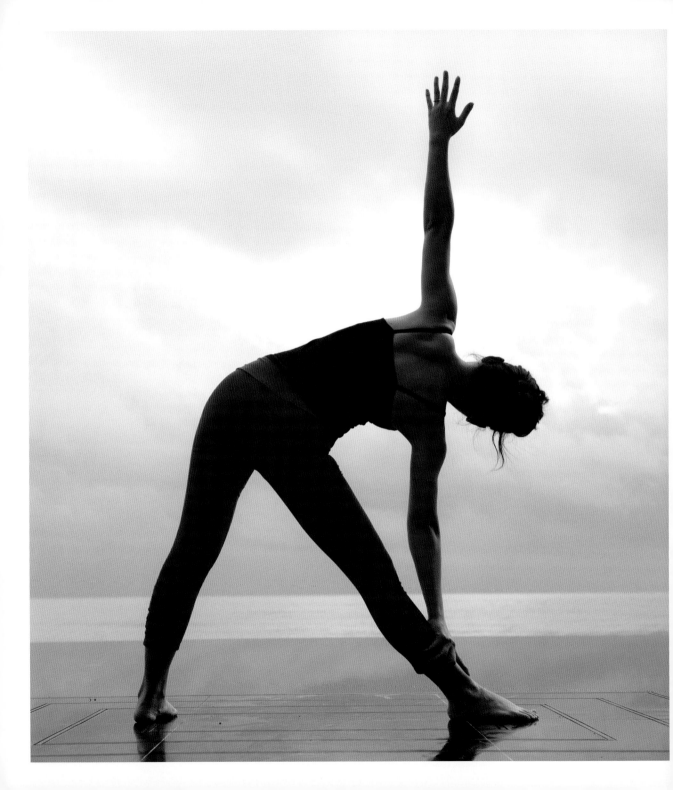

Practitioners like Tracy B., a mom from Fullerton, California, say that marijuana actually helps with focus by calming the unnecessary thoughts and "noise" that otherwise interrupt the meditative process. "Without cannabis I find my mind wandering to the shopping list, what time I need to pick up my daughter from band practice, a difficult client, and a million other chores. When I use marijuana, first I can relax, let it all go, focus on my breathing, and just be in the moment," she says.

To be sure, not everyone is on board the 420 yoga bandwagon. Many practitioners, especially purists who have devoted their lives to the practice of yoga, feel that anything that changes perception inhibits one's ability to experience the true inner self.

Those more open to experimenting, however, could benefit. One word of advice when combining marijuana and yoga: Pay attention to the strain. You may find it difficult to achieve the calm focus necessary for yoga on a strong sativa. On the other end of the spectrum, too strong an indica might just put you to sleep before class is over.

As of now, most 420 yoga classes are offered on the down low. Make inquiries and keep an eye out; as acceptance grows, more of these classes will start coming out of the cannabis closet.

BUDDING BEAUTY

Can marijuana skin products improve the quality of your skin? It depends on the individual product and how it's made, but, when you consider the fact that cannabis is loaded with vitamins, minerals, and antioxidants that can be easily absorbed through the pores of the skin, it would only make sense.

Science shows cannabinoids like CBD and THC can be absorbed through the skin, so in addition to excellent nourishing and moisturizing qualities, topical cannabis products also have the potential to deliver medicinal benefits like reduced inflammation.

Even though the cannabis beauty industry is still in its infancy, you can already find a wide variety of products like moisturizers, lip balms, toners, facial masks, and more, all infused with marijuana. These products will not make you high, yet you will not be able to legally buy them in states where marijuana is illegal. That's right, you could be arrested for using skin cream!

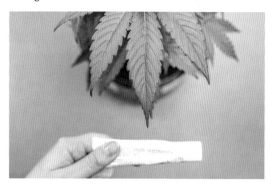

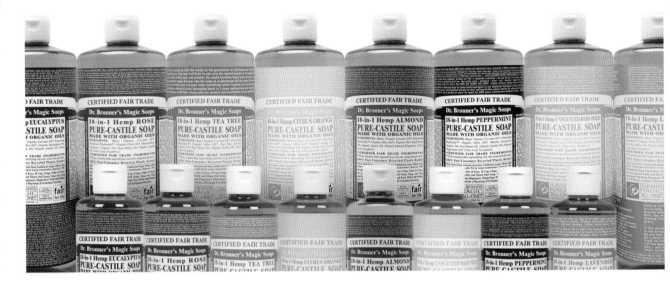

GOTTA HAVE IT! DR. BRONNER'S MAGIC SOAPS

People have been singing the praises of Dr. Bronner's all-natural castile soap since 1948 when Dr. Emanuel Bronner, a third-generation master soap maker, first began to manufacture soap based on formulas he brought from his native Germany. Renowned for their quality, versatility, and eco-friendliness, Dr. Bronner's soap sales exploded in the 1960s with the prolific label messaging urging soap consumers to "realize our transcendent unity across religious and ethnic divides." Hemp oil was added as a superfatting agent in 2000.

Dr. Bronner's Magic Soaps are the number-one-selling natural brand of soap in North America. Today the fourth and fifth generations of the Bronner family run the company and, in addition to the traditional all-vegetable, biodegradable, liquid soap, have added a host of other high-quality, sustainably made organic hemp oil health and beauty products.

Since they're made with hemp, not marijuana, Dr. Bronner's products are readily available everywhere. Consumers can feel good about supporting this progressive company because, in addition to producing high-quality organic products, it invests significant energy and financial resources in worthwhile charities and causes, especially hemp legalization, GMO labeling, and fair trade practices. In fact, over the last five years, Dr. Bronner's spending on social and environmental causes and charities has roughly matched the company's total after-tax income, and they intend to keep it that way (www.drbronner.com).

MARIJUAHHHHHHHHNA: MARY JANE GOES TO THE SPA

A trend still on the down low but gaining popularity, especially in recreationally legal states, are 420-friendly spas. The trend is being spurred on by a growing number of massage therapists who found that the anti-inflammatory properties of massage oils and lotions infused with marijuana not only ease their clients' aches and pains, but also help the therapists' own hands and body keep up with the rigorous physical demands of their profession.

Even though the relaxing topical products will not get you high and won't cause you to fail a drug test, they still remain illegal at the federal level, and spa owners have to deal with a lot of legal red tape in order to offer them. But as the law catches up with public opinion, get ready for marijuana-infused bath salts, oils, and moisturizers, as well as wraps, massages, and more using these products. One enterprising company, Foria, has even started marketing a cannabis-laced personal lubricant. At this rate we'll soon be seeing raw cannabis juice bars and vaping lounges adjacent to the massage rooms and steam baths.

RECIPE FOR A GOOD NIGHT'S SLEEP

Here's a nightcap that's easy to make and sure to help you get your beauty rest, especially when made with indica kief or hash. Gianduja, the classic Italian combination of chocolate and hazelnuts, is even better when ganja gets into the mix. (For daytime, make with a sativa-dominant strain and add a shot of hot espresso to the mix for a caffeinated mocha version.)

Ganjanduja Hot Chocolate
MAKES 1 SERVING

- 1¼ cups milk
- 3 tablespoons chocolate hazelnut spread such as Nutella
- ½ ounce dark chocolate
- ⅛ to ¼ gram decarboxylated kief or powdered hash
- whipped cream for garnish, optional

Combine all ingredients, except for whipped cream, in a small saucepan over medium-low heat. Heat, stirring constantly, until the liquid is scalding but not boiling. Pour into a mug and garnish with whipped cream if desired.

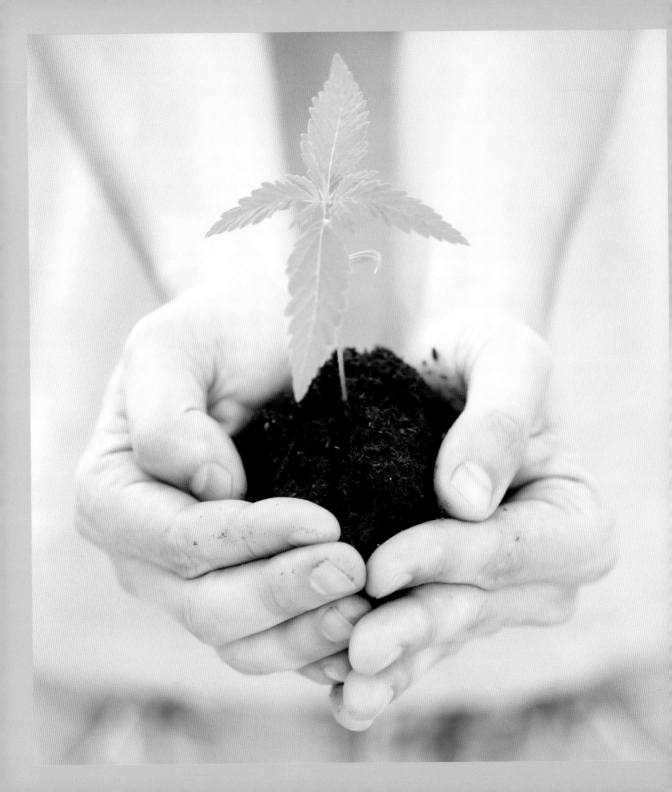

CHAPTER 8
FARMER JANE: GROW *your* OWN

Growing marijuana doesn't take much beyond the basics. Your plants need air, water, light, and nutrients. But how you provide your plants with these elements is where the art of growing premium marijuana comes into play.

If you love to garden, growing marijuana might be for you. Besides the obvious substantial economic savings of growing something yourself—instead of spending up to hundreds of dollars for an ounce—harvesting your own plants offers a number of other benefits:

Purity. If you are a patient, or growing for someone who is, you can be sure what is (or isn't) going into your medicine if you grow it yourself.

Variety. If your favorite strain is hard to find at your regular dispensary or dealer, you can always keep it on hand by growing your own. If you have friends who also grow, you can arrange to grow different strains and swap with each other so you all have variety in your personal stashes.

Satisfaction and stress release. Ask any marijuana gardener—outdoor or indoor—and she'll say the time she spends with her plants is relaxing and reduces stress while providing her with a profound sense of accomplishment and satisfaction.

Profit. I do not recommend that you illegally grow or sell marijuana, but many who do make an excellent living. Others end up in prison, at least as of this writing. Weigh the risks for yourself.

ESSENTIAL GROW TERMS

Whether you decide to grow or not, understanding the world of cannabis gardening will add another volume to your marijuana vocabulary.

Use the words *clones* (most common), *cuts*, or *cuttings* interchangeably to refer to small segments taken from a cannabis plant that are subsequently encouraged to take root in order to grow whole new plants with identical characteristics to the one that donated the *cutting*. The process of *cloning* should be done when the donor plant is in the *vegetative* or *veg* state, meaning it hasn't begun to develop buds. You can opt to take *cuttings* from a veg state plant before you allow it to go into *flowering* or *flower* state—the period of growth when it will develop buds covered in sticky trichomes—or you can alternately choose to keep a single *mother plant* in a state of perpetual veg, ready to donate cuts at any time.

You may also choose to start your plants from *seeds*. If you have friends who grow, see if they will share or sell you seeds. If you live in a state where growing is legal, your favorite dispensary can likely supply you with seeds. If not, there are any number of reliable places on the Internet, usually located in the Netherlands, that discreetly do so, despite the illegality of buying and selling marijuana seeds there, here, and everywhere. In addition to providing an enormous selection of cannabis strains, these sites will let you know what to expect when growing each variety, including how long to wait before harvest, whether the strain thrives better indoors or outdoors, and what to expect from the finished product.

Seed dealers will also offer *feminized seeds*. Because growers are always looking for *sinsemilla* (seed-free female plants), feminized seeds increase but do not guarantee the chance of getting potent girls rather than male plants that typically need to be discarded.

If you opt to grow inside, you can grow in *soil* or use a *hydroponic* system that keeps the roots wet without any dirt being involved at all. An *aeroponic* system will keep roots moist but not submerged.

Growing *organically*—without any chemical nutrients or pesticides—is easier in soil because organic nutrients can clog hydroponic lines. Some growers opt to grow *veganically*, meaning they eschew the use of all animal products such as bat guano or worm castings.

Growers will always want to *flush* their plants—to give them pure water without any nutrients—for about two weeks before harvest. This will purify the plant cells, making for smoother, better-tasting cannabis. You'll also avoid any chemical sensitivity issues when ingesting the marijuana.

THINGS TO CONSIDER BEFORE GOING FORWARD

You can increase your chances of success by working out the details before you begin.

- Will you grow indoors or outdoors? If you do decide to grow indoors, see the additional considerations listed below.

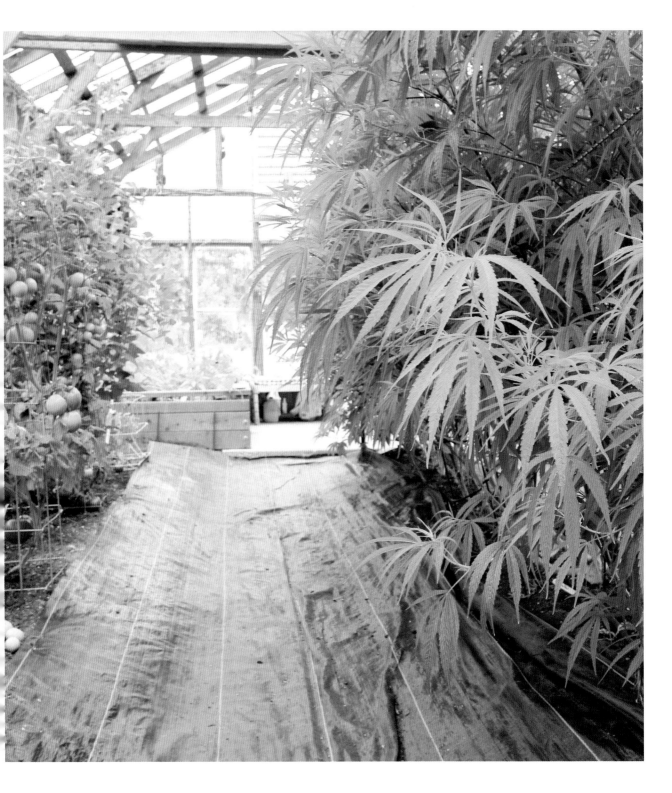

- Do you have a safe, secure place to grow, away from children and nosy neighbors?

- What type of marijuana or strains will you grow? Generally speaking, indicas or indica-dominant hybrids are easier than sativas for beginners to grow and have the added benefits of shorter flowering times and higher yields. Of course, there are countless exceptions to this generalization.

- Do you have the necessary time to see the grow through to completion? If you grow outdoors, figure on working from May through November in addition to preparing soil and starting clones in advance. Indoors, it varies. Indicas will generally need eight to ten weeks in flowering mode, sativas twelve to fourteen weeks. How long you keep plants in veg is up to you, but know that the longer you veg, the bigger your plants will get, so pay attention if your space is limited. Expect your plants to double or more in size after transitioning to a flowering light cycle and before harvest.

STAYING IN VERSUS GOING OUT

If you decide to grow your own marijuana, one of the first decisions you'll have to make is whether to grow inside or outside.

Before we get into the fine print, know that you can grow some decent outdoor weed in a portable pot or two on a balcony, in a discreet spot that gets plenty of sunlight. However, your plants will not get enough light sitting inside on a sunny windowsill. Of course, if you don't have discreet sunny outdoor space, the decision may be made for you.

Outdoor Pros

- Less expensive. You can grow some respectable marijuana with an investment of $100 or less, depending on what you already have on hand. Furthermore, the sun will never send you an exorbitant electric bill.

- Less work/hassle. You will have to watch and tend to your plants, but outdoor grows usually require less maintenance and tinkering.

- More environmentally sound. When you use natural sunlight and rainwater, you demand far less from the environment.

- Bigger harvests. It's hard to beat natural sunlight! Under the best circumstances, you can grow some monster plants outdoors. A friend of mine once took 5 pounds of trimmed flowers from a single outdoor plant!

Outdoor Cons

- Exposed/more vulnerable to humans. Unless you live on a huge plot of land in the middle of nowhere, outdoor grows are generally harder to hide and more exposed. Law enforcement aside, your outdoor grow is prime prey for neighborhood punks, unethical meter readers, or anyone else who likes marijuana and decides to rip you off after spotting your plants. And someone who doesn't like marijuana may report you to the police.

- Exposed/more vulnerable to pests. I'm not saying you can't get predatory pests indoors, but some of the outdoor variety can be difficult, if not impossible, to control. For instance, spider mites are a common problem both inside and out, but you won't have to deal with critters like squirrels, birds, deer, and locusts (yes, locusts) if you grow inside. Remember, all these creatures have endocannabinoid systems too, and they all enjoy cannabis.

- Exposed/more vulnerable to the elements. A week of cloudy days, powerful winds, out-of-season frost and/or excessive heat, or a freak hailstorm can all damage or wipe out your outdoor cannabis crop without warning.

- Only one chance. With an outdoor grow, you get a single shot. If something goes wrong and it dies during the season, you are out of luck until next year.

Indoor Pros

- More controllable. You are God to your indoor plants. You control their water, light, and nutrients; by changing their light cycles you control how long they stay in veg state and when they go into flower; and finally you determine when they are ready for harvest.

- Year-round harvests. You can set up your indoor plants on a rotating schedule so you are continually harvesting throughout the year. Some growers set up to harvest a few plants every week, others every two weeks, and others every month. If you plan to keep a perpetual grow, find a rhythm that works for you.

- Less exposed. In theory, it's easier to hide an indoor grow, unlike an outdoor garden that's exposed to the neighbors.

Indoor Cons

- Way more expensive. Even if you grow in dirt, you will still need a system of lights to grow indoors. To keep the room at optimum temperature, you will probably have to install vents and/or air conditioning, especially if you live in a hot climate. You will want fans to keep the air moving, help strengthen the plants' leaves, and reduce odor. A system to supplement the room's CO_2 content will help you grow better plants with bigger yields. If you don't have a room or two you can dedicate to growing, you'll need to purchase a grow tent or two. It all adds up. Even on the cheap, expect to spend $500 to $2,500 to set up a small indoor grow.

- More work/time-consuming. Indoor grows, especially hydroponic grows, generally take more daily work and tinkering than their outdoor counterparts.

- Bigger learning curve. It's not difficult, but there is more to learn.

- Bigger physical risk. Grow lights use a lot of electricity, possibly risking electrical fires. Always consult a trusted electrician and be sure you have adequate power to handle the electrical drain of your indoor grow. This shouldn't be a problem with one or two plants, but always do your homework before planting.

- Vulnerable to power outages—If you live in an area that's subject to frequent power outages, they can interfere with your plant's light cycle and damage your crop unless you have a generator or other backup that keeps the lights on without interruption.

If you do plan to grow indoors, work out these additional details before proceeding:

- Do you have enough secure space that will not be disturbed to grow indoors? When your plants are in the flowering stage—meaning twelve hours of light and twelve hours of darkness—you cannot go into the room and turn on the lights during dark time. I am not kidding. Your plants will suffer if you do. If you plan to keep plants growing perpetually, you will need separate spaces for plants in both vegetative and flowering states, as each requires a different light cycle—eighteen to twenty-four hours of light a day for veg and twelve hours of light a day for flowering.

- What strain or strains will you grow? Different strains will mature at varying rates—check with your supplier or a reputable Internet source for the type(s) of marijuana you want to grow to be sure they will be compatible in the same garden. Indicas generally take eight to twelve weeks in flowering stage, whereas sativas can take twelve to fourteen weeks.

- Do you have an adequate electrical supply to safely power the necessary lights and equipment? For example, you will need a minimum of 10 amps for a medium-size six-plant grow using up to a 1,000-watt metal halide light for flowering and 200-watt fluorescent lights in the veg room, plus fans and other miscellaneous electronics.

- Do you have enough money to pay the substantially increased power bill you will be incurring?

- Will anyone in the house or nearby be disturbed by the pungent aroma of growing marijuana, and, if so, have you planned for an air filtration system?

SEX IN THE GARDEN

Unless you want to specifically breed marijuana plants in order to harvest seeds, you'll want to grow ONLY female plants. If you took a clone or cutting from another female plant, you're guaranteed another girl. If you are growing from seeds, how do you know if your

GOTTA HAVE IT!
Portable Grow Tents

Undoubtedly the easiest way to set up a small indoor personal grow room is with a grow tent. An Internet search will yield lots of different examples of these mylar tents specifically made for the purpose of growing marijuana. The tents have places for hanging lights; they zip closed to be light-tight; and they have openings where you can attach ventilation. Grow tents can fit in almost any unused corner or large closet and can be deconstructed when not in use. If you don't want to or don't have the space to build an indoor grow room, a portable grow tent can provide a quick and easy out-of-the-box solution.

plants are male or female? You have to learn how to "sex" them.

In an outdoor garden, start to look for signs of sex in late June when the days begin to get shorter. In an indoor grow, start looking a week or two after transitioning your plants from their vegetative state of eighteen to twenty-four hours a day of light to a cycle of twelve hours of light and twelve of darkness, which will propel them into "plant puberty."

Look carefully and closely at the plant nodes, the places where two tiny branches come together. The male plants will have small, round, testicle-like nodes here, while the female nodes will more closely resemble

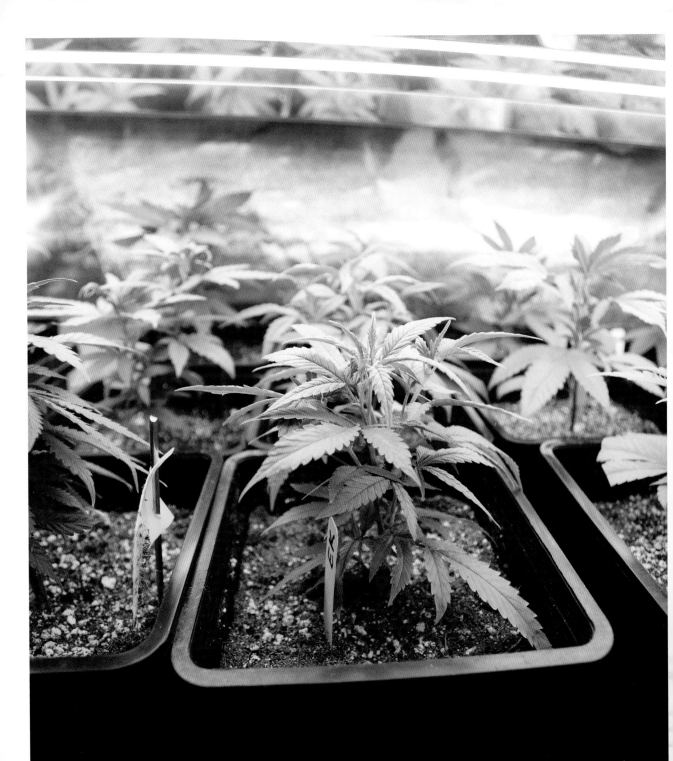

HERMAPHRODITES

On rare occasions, marijuana plants exhibit both male and female characteristics. I have yet to personally see a *hermaphrodite* (growers also call them *Hermies*) in one of my gardens, but professional cultivator friends tell me they happen more frequently when growing from feminized seeds, although they're still rare. If you ever find a hermaphrodite plant, it needs to get pulled along with the males as it can pollinate itself along with the girls and ruin the entire grow.

a vaginal opening, albeit one surrounded by feathery tendrils.

It may take some practice, but once you see the difference you'll be able to quickly sex your plants. You'll need to kill all your male plants before they begin to mature. I know, how cold-blooded. But even a single male can pollinate all your beautiful girls, and if that happens all their energy will go toward producing seeds instead of trichomes. What a waste!

TROUBLESHOOTING

I polled some grower friends about the most common mistakes made by new marijuana gardeners. Here are some things you should take care to avoid.

- Overwatering. Your plants need plenty of moisture but be sure not to drown them.

- Too many nutrients. Again, the plants need nutrients, but too much of a good thing will harm them.

- Too much manhandling. Marijuana plants are hardy, but too much handling can break stems and damage them long before they get to harvest.

- Letting light in. When you grow indoors, the plants need to stay in complete darkness during their dark periods. Opening the door or turning on the lights—even for a minute—can disrupt the plant's natural cycles.

- Failing to notice pests. Use magnifying glasses to carefully examine your plants at frequent intervals. Pests like spider mites are easy to miss if you're not paying attention. The earlier you catch pest problems, the better your chances of saving the crop.

- Harvesting too soon. Patience, please. Wait for the proper moment to get the best results (see page 90).

HOW TO:

A Little Extra Free Insurance

Sadly, even in states that have legalized marijuana for medicinal use, law enforcement and prosecutors frequently take a dim view of cultivators, especially if they suspect you are making a profit from the grow. You can give yourself some low-cost insurance by putting labels with some variation of the following on all your plants, pots, equipment, and anything else in the room that might potentially be considered evidence:

- *Medical Marijuana grown in strict compliance with [identify your state's medical marijuana laws by statute number here].*

In any state, legal or not, include

- *"Jury Nullification: Jurors have the right to vote not guilty on immoral laws."*

In addition, prominently display a copy of your doctor's recommendation that allows you to legally use medical marijuana in several places in the grow room. If you are a caregiver growing for other patients, make sure copies of their doctors' recommendations are also on obvious display.

Why? Because in federal cases you will always be denied an "affirmative defense," meaning the judge will not allow the jury to hear a single word about legal medical marijuana (remember, cannabis is illegal at the federal level). Some prohibitionist judges have even denied affirmative defenses in state cases.

But if you have labels and doctor's recommendations on PROMINENT display, you will force the jury to hear about medical marijuana and their right to nullify laws they find unjust, whether the judge or prosecutor wants them to or not. The prosecution's only other option is to not use photos of your grow room as evidence against you at all. But the second they put those photos in front of a jury, your attorney can inquire as to exactly what is written on all those labels!

GARDEN SAFETY AND SECURITY

The biggest predatory threat to your marijuana garden aren't aphids, spider mites, or locusts. The biggest predators are . . . human beings. Of course you'll want to avoid the attention of law enforcement, but it goes way beyond that. Because of prohibition, the cash value of your marijuana garden will be substantially more than, say, an equally impressive haul of tomatoes. Therefore, you are always at risk of getting ripped off. Implement these tips and keep yourself and your garden as safe as possible.

- The first rule of Cannabis Gardening Club is that you don't talk about Cannabis Gardening Club. Keep your garden on a strictly need-to-know basis.

Do not go bragging about it to your friends. Remember that every person who knows about your garden increases your exposure because you never know whom those people will tell.

- Never post proud pictures of your plants on social media. Yes, people do it all the time and don't have a problem, but why take the risk? Those photos can come back to haunt you in any number of ways—if you get into legal trouble, if you're involved in a custody dispute, if you're trying to get a job, and more.

- Keep your home in order—pick up the trash, mow the lawn, avoid loud music or too many people coming and going, and so on. In other words, don't give the neighbors any reason to complain about anything and never give the police an excuse to stop by.

- If you grow outdoors, at minimum, keep your garden behind a locked gate. If you grow indoors, keep it in a locked room.

- Don't throw out incriminating trash in your home trash cans—things like empty nutrient bottles, leaves, or roots.

- Make sure grow room windows and doors are light-tight and that light cannot be seen from outside the house.

GOTTA HAVE IT!
Jeweler's Loupe

A jeweler's loupe is essential for determining when your marijuana plants are ready for harvest because it's impossible to tell the color of microscopic trichomes with the naked eye. But gaze through the lens and you'll be transported into an enchanted world of sparkling trichome forests covering the surface of your plants.

You can get an inexpensive loupe for a few dollars, but even the deluxe models with built-in lights shouldn't set you back more than twenty bucks. If you plan to grow, you will need this tool, but even if you don't, you'll find it both fun and fascinating to examine your stash because those same magical trichome forests exist on the stuff you're smoking!

- The larger the grow, the stronger the aroma. Figure out whether others can pick up on the scent of your grow and filter accordingly.

- If you have noisy fans or hydroponic equipment, either find a way to sound-proof the room or come up with a reasonable explanation if any friends get curious. (Never lie to law enforcement, however; instead, refer to Chapter 5).

WELCOME TO THE HARVEST FESTIVAL

Deciding on the right moment to harvest your lovely green ladies is one of the trickiest parts of growing cannabis. I know how it feels to anxiously await a harvest. The tiny seedlings you planted have grown like weeds (yes, pun intended) and are so enormous you just *know* they have to be ready.

Patience, grasshopper. You may *think* they're ready, but you won't be able to know for sure by looking at the plants with the naked eye.

While harvesting too early is one of the most common rookie mistakes, it's not a huge tragedy. If you're a little off, you should still get some decent weed. But if you wait to harvest at the right time, you'll be rewarded with a higher-quality, smoother, more potent final product.

Read the sidebar on page 89 and go get yourself a jeweler's loupe well before your plants should be ready for harvest. Start looking at them early and you will notice that the glistening trichomes, or resinous glands that cover the surface of the leaves and buds, will be clear, resembling tiny crystal mushrooms. As the plants start to get closer to harvest time, the trichomes will become a translucent milky white. Begin to watch carefully when you notice this change. When you start to notice the trichomes taking on an amber color,

you've reached the magic moment—by most people's standards. Chop those babies down and begin the trimming and curing process.

If you let the plants go on longer, the trichomes will take on a deep amber color. By most grower's standards, this is a little late, not that it still won't be potent weed. Some theorize the darker amber the trichomes, the more the marijuana will induce couch-lock. If you like to be so stoned that you can't move from the sofa, harvest accordingly.

To some degree, knowing when to harvest becomes a matter of personal preference. Experiment to discover what you like and keep in mind that different strains will have subtle and sometimes not-so-subtle differences in readiness.

TRIMMING TREATISE

You've chopped down your plants at the stem. Now what? It's time to get to work on trimming and curing.

In my opinion, the easiest time to trim your plants is right after chopping them down. I like to wear latex gloves because the plants are sticky. You can forgo the gloves, but expect your hands to get tacky, as they would if you were handling pine pitch.

Start by gently pulling off all the large fan leaves by their stems and put them aside in a pile. Some folks use these for raw

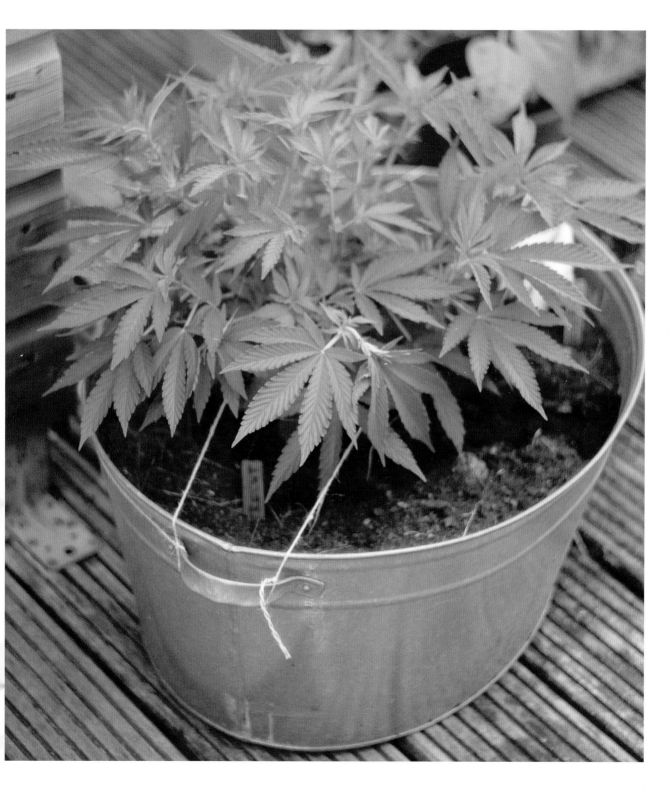

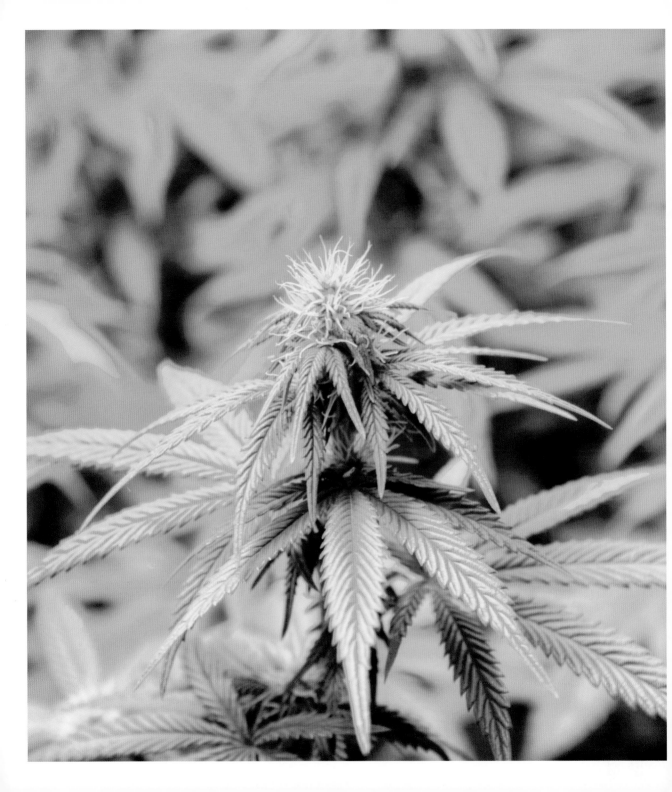

cannabis juicing—an antioxidant-rich liquid that puts wheatgrass to shame. You can also use them for making cannabis-infused butter or oil, although you'll need to use far more than you would of the tiny sugar leaves close to the buds or flowers themselves. While you can technically use fan leaves for making hash and other concentrates too (see Chapter 3), I don't because I find that the plant material–to–trichome ratio is not conducive to high-quality concentrates.

I recommend trimming the plant while keeping the buds on the stems because it is easier and more space-efficient to dry and cure in this form. Simply use a clothespin to attach the stems to wire coat hangers. Some buds may come off in the process. That's fine. Set them aside and cure them in a single layer on a wire baking rack.

Now take your scissors and carefully "give the buds a haircut," or trim off all the small leaves surrounding the bud, taking care to avoid cutting into the flower itself. If you have a hard time, just get close now; you can always manicure further after curing when you remove the flowers from the stalks.

Some people take an enormous amount of time to trim their plants. If you plan on entering any competitions, or if you demand top dollar for your gardening wares from marijuana dispensaries, expect to do so as well. When I'm trimming for my own personal use,

however, I'm not nearly as precise. The tiny sugar leaves have tons of trichomes on them and I don't mind if a few stay in the mix.

Save all your trimmings for either cooking or making concentrates. Waste not, want not.

After you have grown a few different strains, you'll find some are far easier to trim than others. Some plants can be almost entirely trimmed using nothing but your fingers to pull off the leaves. Others have so many tiny leaves and branches they take hours of careful scissor work.

Tips for Trimmers

- Invest in a decent pair of small, ergonomic, spring-loaded scissors designed for gripping and squeezing. Those with slightly curved blades make it easier to trim around the buds.

- Latex gloves will keep your hands from getting sticky.

- Have some 92-percent-or-higher-grade alcohol on hand for periodically cleaning scissors and hands while trimming.

- Avoid repetitive stress injury while trimming by frequently taking breaks and taking time to stretch your hands.

- Resin known as *scissor hash* will begin to collect on gloves, hands, and scissors, although it's technically kief since it hasn't been heated and pressed (see Chapter 3). Carefully scrape it off and use it for smoking or cooking. To easily remove the sticky resin from gloves, stick them in the freezer for 15 minutes or so. Remove gloves from freezer and then vigorously rub them over a sheet of white paper to collect the falling concentrate.

THE PERFECT CURE

Well-cured marijuana produces a smoother, more flavorful smoke or vape experience. Many inexperienced growers have ruined countless excellent marijuana crops during the curing phase, so don't ignore this last essential step.

What you are trying to accomplish is to remove the moisture from the flowers without making them brittle and dry as a bone.

Too much moisture and you risk moldy flowers. Trust me, I know from experience that nothing is as heartbreaking as a big, beautiful jar of marijuana buds covered in fuzzy white mold. You do not want to smoke or eat that, so in the garbage they go. Let your plants get too dry and they will crumble to dust when you touch them.

Take the trimmed marijuana stalks and hang them in a cool, dark, well-ventilated place. Think of it as a root cellar; ideally the temperature should be in the 60s, but you may have to work with what you've got. You want moisture to evaporate, but not too quickly. A circulating fan or two can help the process. After a few days—the amount of time will vary due to external factors as well as the amount of moisture in your particular plants—you can cut the flowers off the stem and place them in glass jars. You'll know it's time when the buds feel dry to the touch on the surface, but the branches don't yet snap off like dry twigs.

Don't pack the buds too tightly because you'll need room to stir the mix. Seal the jars and keep in a cool, dark, dry place. At least once a day, open the jars and stir the flowers inside. If moisture has accumulated, leave the jars open for several hours to overnight before sealing again and repeating the process. After about two weeks, all the moisture should be gone and you're left with perfectly cured marijuana that is ready to smoke or vape.

Curing Tips

- Especially if you live in a place where you need to be discreet, don't underestimate how pungent the aroma of curing cannabis can be. A charcoal exhaust filter in the curing space can help eliminate olfactory clues.

- The climate where you live can affect how the plants cure: Too much moisture in the air will lengthen the process; too little moisture and things can dry too quickly on the surface while retaining moisture in the center. Even altitude can make a difference. I grew (indoors) and cured at 7,000 feet. What seemed like perfectly cured marijuana quickly transformed into fluffy, wet, undercured cannabis during the hour-long drive down the mountain to sea level.

- If you've let your weed get too dry, you might be able to reverse it. Seal it in a jar with a small piece of barely moist paper towel. Leave it for a day and then check it out; it might be just fine. If necessary, stir and give it another day or two. Remove the paper towel when the weed no longer feels bone dry and brittle. Take care to check at least once a day because it can grow mold if left too long.

SAFETY PATROL:
Kids, Guns, and Grows

No, I am not going to lecture you about keeping guns out of the hands of your children. I am going to assume you are smart enough to already have that under control. But know that if you are growing marijuana and have either—children or guns—in the house, the potential consequences of a bust go way up. If all three are present, you'd better have a good attorney.

Any time guns and drugs are found together, expect extra charges. If your children are around a grow, regardless of the absence or presence of weapons, you risk not only child endangerment charges, but the possibility of having Child Protective Services remove the children and place them in foster care and, in the worst-case scenario, up for adoption.

Ironically, this will NOT happen if you have children and guns in your home but no marijuana.

Don't think living in a legal or quasilegal state makes these risks go away. If you have underage kids or guns—even legally permitted guns—in the house, think twice before growing cannabis.

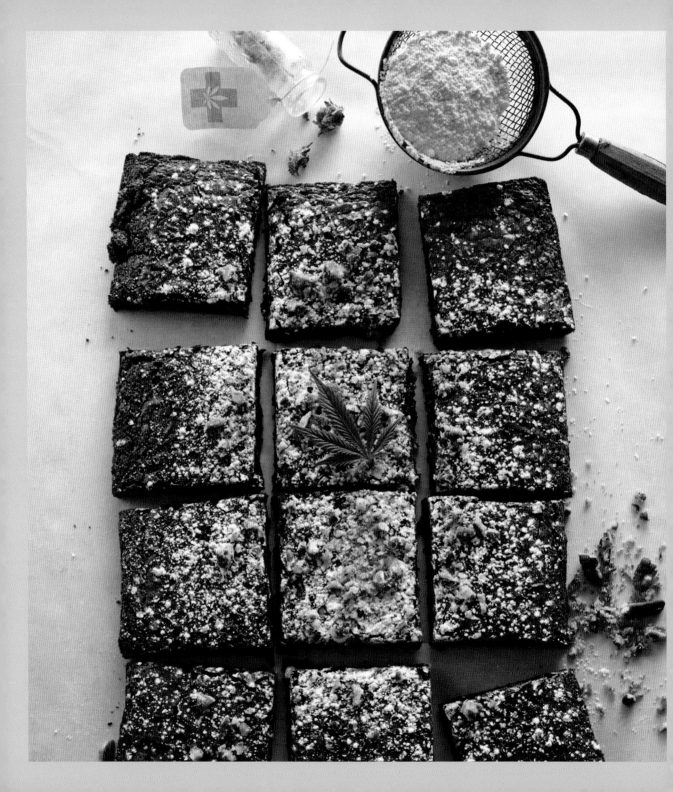

CHAPTER 9

STIRRING *the* POT: COOKING *with* CANNABIS

Peruse the wares offered at your average marijuana dispensary and you will find shelves and refrigerators filled with a cornucopia of medicated desserts. But you'll be hard-pressed to find anything savory, let alone healthy. The lack of alternatives to sweet edibles has been bemoaned on many panels about edible marijuana I have served on, and the public consistently asks for more choices every year. Ironically, when I converse with collective managers, they claim that savory and healthy fare just doesn't sell.

Of course, whenever you mention edible cannabis, most people instantly think of brownies, as if that's the only food that can carry the magical properties of marijuana. While there is nothing wrong with brownies, there's a whole world of cannabis cooking beyond them. In fact, you can "cannabinize" nearly any recipe.

Besides a wider variety of culinary choices, making your own marijuana-infused foods offers other enticing benefits:

Discretion. Unlike smoking or even vaporizing, edible cannabis provides a completely discreet way of ingestion. You are the only one who needs to know. Just be sure to eat where nobody is going to ask you to share . . . unless you brought enough for everyone.

Longer lasting. While the effects of smoked or vaporized marijuana come on immediately, the effects of edible cannabis last longer, three to four hours or more.

Smoke-free. Some people just don't like to smoke. Period. Others have medical conditions that contraindicate smoking. Edibles to the rescue!

Control. Commercial edibles are usually made from a *salad*, or a mixture of different cannabis strains, so you never know what you

EDIBLE MEDIBLES

Edibles and *medibles* are two interchangeable terms in the cannabis industry that refer to foods infused with marijuana. In a more casual setting, if a stoner ever goes out of his way to tell you that a particular food is *tainted* or *leaded*, he isn't saying it's unsafe to eat, but rather that it contains cannabis.

are going to get. When you make your own, you can incorporate the type of marijuana that works best for you into the kinds of foods you like to eat.

Customized dosing. Someday all commercial edibles will be reliably lab tested and labeled. Then, cannabis consumers will be able to know, in advance, what kind of dose to expect. Unfortunately, right now this is the exception rather than the rule, so consumers typically take their chances and hope for the best. I've eaten many a commercial medible that had no effect whatsoever, and I've had a few that almost knocked me out (figuratively speaking). When you make your own, Goldilocks, you get a medible that is just right for you.

More effective for certain ailments. Medical marijuana patients dealing with chronic pain, neurological pain, and insomnia tend to especially benefit from the edible form of THC delivery.

Frugal. Providing you grow your own, you almost can't afford not to cook with the leaves and trimmings that would otherwise be discarded (unless you plan on making hash, in which case you should turn to Chapter 3).

WHAT TO EXPECT: SMOKING OR VAPING VERSUS EATING

You can ingest THC by smoking, vaping, and eating marijuana, and all these methods will offer therapeutic benefits, and all will get you high (see Chapter 2). But there are some important differences.

Metabolism. Inhaled marijuana enters the body through the lungs. Edible marijuana is metabolized by the liver, which leads us to the next point.

Speed of onset. When you inhale marijuana via smoking or vaporizing it, you feel the results almost instantly. When you digest cannabis, it will take at least 30 minutes and as much as an hour and a half or longer before you feel the effects.

Duration of effects. The effects of inhaled cannabis dissipate relatively quickly. An hour or less after smoking, most, if not all, of the effect will have worn off. With edibles, the effects can last for several hours. Effects will usually completely dissipate in about four hours but occasionally can last longer.

Dosing. It's easy to get just the right amount of inhaled marijuana. When you feel high, you stop. That's the end of it until you smoke more. The strength of edibles can vary widely, even if similar plant material was used to make them. Furthermore, because it takes so long to take effect, people often think edibles aren't "working" and eat more, resulting in overmedication (more on that later in this chapter).

Intensity. Edible marijuana is thought to be stronger than smoked because of the way it is metabolized through the liver, and also because some of the THC is burned off during smoking. Since combustion never occurs when making edibles, more THC actually goes into the food and likewise into your body.

Side effects. Regardless of how it is taken, the most commonly reported side effect of using marijuana, aside from mild euphoria, is what some call "cotton mouth" (dry mouth in medical terms). This unfortunate but not serious side effect tends to be more pronounced with edibles than combustibles.

Conditional effects. Certain medical conditions such as insomnia and chronic pain tend to respond especially well to edible marijuana. For some patients it is not necessary to have a psychoactive dose in order to receive benefit. In fact, for pain management, many patients eat small amounts throughout the

SAFETY PATROL:

When Segregation Is a Good Thing

Whether you make your own edibles or purchase them, make sure they are always clearly labeled and keep them away from other foods in order to avoid them accidentally falling into the wrong hands, or surprising someone who was not expecting to eat medicated foods. This is especially important if children are in the house.

day in order to keep a baseline dose in their system without ever feeling high!

WHAT KIND OF MARIJUANA SHOULD I COOK WITH?

You can cook with anything from leaves and trimmings all the way up to the finest pure buds.

Those who grow their own typically cook with trimmings and leaves in order to put those otherwise wasted parts of the plant to practical use. Most people who aren't growing generally cook with low-quality shake or low-quality bud because marijuana is expensive and those options are often more economical. True connoisseurs, those for whom money is no object, or growers who are so flush with product they have more than they'll ever use (it happens), cook with high-quality bud.

All these options will get you high. Some of the most powerful edibles I have created were made with leaves and trimmings, albeit leaves and trimmings from a high-quality plant. My point is that potency can be achieved from any decent plant matter, or even any medium or fair- to low-quality plant matter, if you use enough of it.

So why might you use top-shelf weed for cooking? For one thing, you'll need less of it than you would of shake, trimmings, or lower-quality bud. There's also an interesting intersection of cannabis and foodie culture that happens here, with true foodies and cannophiles matching flavors of foods and marijuana strains much as sommeliers match foods with wine. If you aren't such a connoisseur, you will probably opt to cook with less expensive herb.

Keep in mind that more expensive plant material does not necessarily mean better cooking material. There's a saying in the marijuana industry, "Smell sells," referring to the fact that consumers tend to favor tight, pretty buds with a pungent aroma. Savvy cannabis consumers should also know that testing laboratories have found these qualities do not correlate with a product's potency. While nice-smelling marijuana might provide a more enjoyable smoke, there is no reason for the cannabis cook to pay for this "benefit,"

as it will be wasted in the process of creating edibles.

The best kind of marijuana to use in your cooking is the kind that works best for you. The number of cannabis strains now available boggles the mind. It will take experimentation with lots of different strains to find the ones that work best for you (oh, darn!). Different strains affect people in different ways. A variety that makes one person feel energetic and euphoric might make another feel paranoid or anxious. Your personal smoking notes (see Chapter 1) can help you here. Chances are if you liked smoking or vaping it, you'll like cooking with it too. If you're lucky enough to have access to a quality dispensary, a knowledgeable budtender can help you out as well.

If you're not so lucky, choose by marijuana type: indica, sativa, or hybrid (again, see Chapter 1). Most strains these days are hybrids, but they will be indica- or sativa-dominant. If you don't know which exact strain will work well for you, choose by one of these broad categories. Think of them as the equivalent of red, white, and rosé in wine, under which there are many varieties and variations.

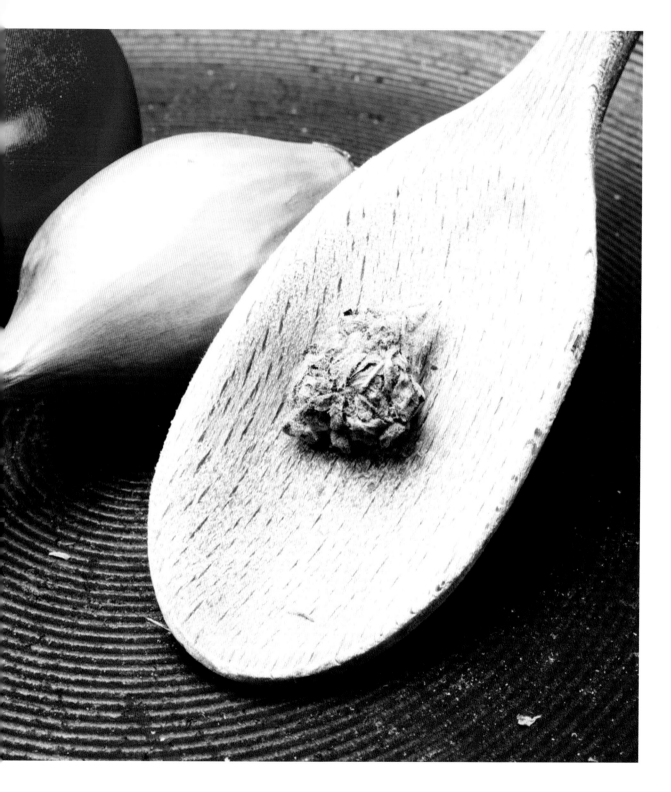

HOW TO PREPARE MARIJUANA FOR COOKING

You'll want to cook with cured, dried marijuana, not fresh green plants. Prepare plant material by making sure all large stems and stalks are removed.

There is no need to grind the plant material in a blender, food processor, or coffee grinder, despite the hordes of websites, blogs, and even a commercially available marijuana butter–making appliance that recommend doing so. The parts of the plant you want to infuse into your butter or oil are the trichomes, or resin glands, and those are ON the plants, not IN them. So grinding your weed to a fine pulp serves no practical purpose. In fact, doing so makes it more difficult to remove the plant material during straining and will infuse your foods with more of that green herbal flavor most of us are trying to avoid.

If you find you have more dried plant material than you can cook with right away, store it in a well-sealed plastic bag in the freezer until you're ready. The cold temperature prevents the growth of mold and also helps maintain the marijuana's potency over time.

HOW MUCH TO USE

It is impossible for anyone to make a definitive recommendation about the amount of cannabis a given dish needs to be effective. Far too many variables come into play.

By their nature cannabis recipes, including the ones in this book, must include an amount of marijuana to use. But the cook must always understand that these amounts are only rough guidelines.

Before we get into the process of determining exactly how much marijuana to use in our cooking, there are some important key points that need to be understood. All cannabis is not created equal! The same amounts of different strains of marijuana will NOT be equal in potency.

Just because you have cooked with a given strain in the past does not mean that you will know the strength of the food made from the same strain from a different source. Testing laboratories show wide ranges in potency within the same strain, depending on where and how it was grown. Even home growers who use the same techniques and nutrients, and start with clones from the same mother plant, may expect variations from crop to crop.

Not to worry. People have been managing to successfully dose their marijuana edibles for thousands of years without the benefit of testing labs. By experimenting with the tips and techniques contained in this chapter, you will get the knack of knowing how much cannabis to use in your cooking.

Aside from potency, every cannabis strain is different, each containing varying degrees of specific cannabinoids. This is why some strains make you sleepy and others make you energetic. If you are cooking with a new strain, test its potency and effects both before cooking and before eating a normal portion (see sidebar) in order to estimate its strength.

Even though there may be some variations, keeping notes on the strains you cook with has real value. As you become more experienced and try different marijuana strains in edibles, you will find some work better for you than others. Carefully evaluate how you feel after trying each new strain. Does it make you sleepy? Energetic? Euphoric? Paranoid or anxious? Any of these effects can be achieved or mitigated by experimenting with different strains. You can expect similar results when using the same strain in the future, even though the strength of the new plant may or may not be the same.

In addition to the type and quality of the marijuana used in cooking, other variables will affect the strength of the finished edibles:

Size. The weight of the person eating the food will alter how much they feel the medication. Naturally, larger people usually need larger doses than smaller people. I say usually

HOW TO:
Test Edibles for Potency

A quick way to get an indication of the strength of the marijuana *before* cooking with it is to smoke or vaporize a small amount. While cooking will produce a somewhat different and usually stronger effect, smoking or vaporizing will give you a general idea of what to expect in regard to potency.

If you don't know how strong a given batch of cannabis butter, oil, or prepared edibles is—and you usually won't—it's best to test the waters before pigging out. Start with a half portion, or even a quarter portion if you consider yourself a "lightweight." Wait at least an hour and a half. If you feel the effects of the marijuana, don't eat any more. If you don't, try another piece, or alternatively, wait until the next day and try a larger portion. Even if you don't feel a "high," you will still be getting medicinal benefits.

because, again, different individuals have different metabolisms and tolerance levels and likewise react to cannabis in different ways.

Frequency. How regularly and often people use cannabis will affect how much they need to feel the physical effects. The more you use, the greater your tolerance. However, even frequent and heavy cannabis consumers who stop for just a day or two will likely experience a heightened effect the first time they use marijuana again after abstaining.

Hunger. Eating marijuana edibles on an empty stomach will cause you to feel their effect more quickly and profoundly than if you consumed them after eating other foods or in conjunction with other foods.

What do you want? Before adding cannabis to your cooking, consider the desired final outcome. Some people want little, if any, psychotropic effect (believe it or not). Others seek a strong high. Dose accordingly.

Recommended Dosage Ranges

The following chart provides dose ranges for leaf/trim, bud, and concentrates. There is a large range, as you can see, because of the factors we already discussed. The dosage range for concentrates is even wider.

I'll emphasize again that the information below is a general guideline that needs to be weighed against the factors covered above

when determining the amount of cannabis to use in your recipes.

The amounts suggested are for individual servings, for a person who weighs about 150 pounds. If you have a recipe you want to add cannabis to, you'll need to know how many servings the total recipe makes and dose accordingly. Try to determine an amount that seems reasonable for your needs, taking into account the strength of the plant material used and the factors listed above. When you've finished cooking, use the testing techniques described in the How To sidebar on page 110 to assess your dosing skills and adjust the edible's portion size accordingly.

CANNABIS MATERIAL	RECOMMENDED DOSAGE RANGE PER INDIVIDUAL SERVING
Marijuana leaf/trim	½ to 2 grams
Average bud	¼ to 1 gram
High-quality bud	⅛ to ½ gram
Kief or hash or other concentrate	⅛ to 1 grams

FAT IS YOUR FRIEND

In order for the THC in cannabis to metabolize, it needs the presence of fat, alcohol, or glycerin. For our purposes, we need to consider the fat content of foods. If you are cooking with marijuana-infused butter or oil, this step is covered. But when cooking with kief or hash, keep in mind that the recipe needs to contain some fat. It can come in the form of butter or oil, but it doesn't have to. Eggs, cream, whole milk, yogurt, cheeses, meats, tofu, avocados, nuts, and many other foods contain fat. Any of them will help to activate the THC in your recipe. Keep in mind that no one particular type of fat works better than others. Use what works best for the recipe you are preparing.

Dairy products work especially well in cannabis cooking because of the presence of lecithin, an emulsifier that helps bind THC to fat. Vegetarians and vegans should note that lecithin is also present in many milk substitutes, including soy milk and rice milk.

You can medicate fat-free foods, but you will want to consume them along with other foods or drinks that contain some fat in order to gain maximum benefits.

GOTTA HAVE IT!
Slow Cookers

You can make marijuana-infused butter and oils on the stove top, but a slow cooker will make the job soooo much easier, especially if you plan on cooking with cannabis with any regularity. This inexpensive kitchen appliance, which you can also use to make convenient unmedicated meals, offers several advantages over the stovetop method:

- allows you to start cooking and forget about it for hours without having to monitor temperature or water levels.

- allows infusion to occur slowly at a consistent low temperature over a long period of time.

- reduces the amount of odor over stovetop cooking.

The environment can get rather fragrant when cooking with cannabis. If this is a concern for you, Hamilton Beach makes a line of slow cookers called "Stay and Go" that seal and clamp closed in order to make it easy for cooks to transport foods to potluck dinners and parties. While the cannabis cook doesn't necessarily need the clamp function when making butter and oil, the rubber gasket seal on the lid is useful as it seals almost all the odor inside the crock.

Unless you open the lid, there is hardly any smell at all. It works so well that I made a batch of marijuana butter in a "Stay and Go" slow cooker while having a business meeting in the adjoining room. Nobody had a clue until I told them.

MAKING BUTTER AND OIL

Since THC, the psychoactive component of marijuana, is fat-soluble, butter and oil make ideal ways to bond the cannabinoids to food. Likewise, cannabis-infused butter or cooking oils are the backbone of many medicated recipes. With these staples stored in your refrigerator or freezer, you'll be able to make medicated foods anytime.

I've listed the amounts I used to test the recipes in this book below. You can and should alter the suggested amounts to meet your needs, but these guidelines will get you started. You can use more than the recommended amount of cannabis in order to make your butter or oil more concentrated. This has advantages, especially if you are trying to lose weight or cut calories, as the more potent and concentrated your butter or oil, the less of it you'll need to use to achieve a proper dose. On the downside, the more concentrated the fat, the stronger its herbal flavor and green color.

To make about 1 cup of cannabutter, canna-margarine, or infused oils, you will need the following:

- 1¼ cups unsalted butter or margarine, or 1¼ cups cooking oil: olive, vegetable, canola, corn, peanut, or grapeseed. (You can even infuse solid-at-room-temperature fats like coconut oil or vegetable shortening should you choose.)

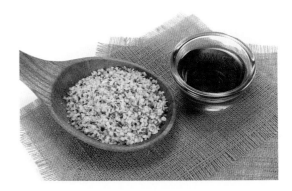

- 1 ounce average- to high-quality trim or low-quality dried bud, or ½ ounce average-quality dried bud.

- About 4 cups water.

Slow cooker method. Add butter or oil, plant material, and water to the slow cooker and cook on low for 6 to 10 hours. Some folks slow-cook their butter for as long as 2 to 3 days. Feel free to do so if you choose, but after testing longer cooking times, I found no improvement in quality or potency. In fact, I noticed a stronger herbal flavor and not much else.

Stovetop method. Place butter or oil, plant material, and water in a large Dutch oven on the stove top. Bring to a boil, reduce heat to very low, and simmer covered for 2 to 4 hours or more. Take care to monitor the liquid level often, adding water as necessary to always keep at least 3 cups in the pot.

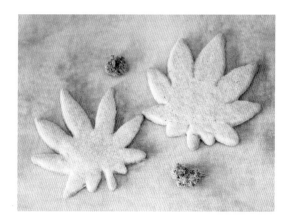

The easiest and most efficient way to separate marijuana-infused oil from water is to use a kitchen gadget called a gravy separator. The unique design of this small pitcher, with the spout on the bottom, allows you to pour out the water while retaining every drop of oil floating at the top. During the holidays, gravy separators are sold everywhere, even supermarkets. Gourmet shops carry them year-round. You can also find extra-large gravy separators at restaurant supply stores.

Why Water?

Without water in the mix, the plant material absorbs too much of the butter and oil. When that happens, usable product will go into the trash, a problem that's reduced when adding water. The increased liquid volume also gives cooks the option to add more plant material in order to make more concentrated infusions if they wish.

Including water in the mix, especially when cooking on the stove top, also ensures the cannabis will never reach a higher temperature than the boiling point of 212 degrees F. Also, the chlorophyll and terpenes—the parts of the plant that give it its flavor and color—are water-soluble, and many of them will likewise bind to water during the cooking process instead of infusing themselves into the fats along with the THC. In practical terms, this means less herbal flavor and green color in the finished marijuana-infused butter or oil.

That said, the butter or oil might still appear plenty green, even when cooked with water. The shade will vary from strain to strain, with some coming out pale green or almost yellow, while others take on a deep forest green color. Keep in mind, however, that color has nothing to do with potency.

DRAIN AND STRAIN

The draining process is identical for stovetop and slow cooker methods. Place a cheesecloth-lined strainer over a large pot or bowl, and strain the liquid through that.

WAIT! Before discarding plant material, pour a large kettle full of boiling water over the full strainer in order to wash through any extra butter or oil clinging to the plant material. Taking the time to do this extra step will increase your yield.

Allow everything to cool and then squeeze out as much liquid as possible from the plant material in the cheesecloth before discarding. Chill the water and oil, or water and liquid butter. The fat will rise to the top. Butter solidifies when cold, making it easy to simply lift the piece off. Rinse the butter chunk with cold, fresh water to remove any cannawater or plant material that might be clinging to it.

Oil will rise to the top of the water but often won't solidify. No problem. You can use a spoon to skim the oil off the water.

Now it's time to strain one more time to remove as much sediment as possible. Place a double layer of cheesecloth over a strainer and pour the oil through. To strain butter, melt it, strain, and then chill again until solid. This second straining is optional, but taking the extra step will give you a cleaner, purer finished product.

Refrigerate infused butter or oil until ready to use, or freeze for even longer storage. Fats can still go rancid in the freezer so try to use within three months.

You're now ready to start cooking with cannabutter and canna-oil!

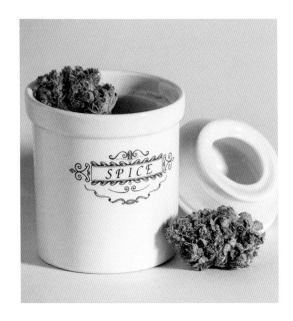

COOKING WITH BUD

Cannabis cooking has come a long way since Alice B. Toklas whipped up batches of her legendary "Haschich Fudge" for Paris's literary elite in the 1920s. While adding pulverized bud to her concoction might have achieved the desired "medicinal" result, today's edible marijuana recipes use techniques that make the cuisine every bit as pleasurable as its aftereffects. Why struggle to choke food down when it can be both medicated and delicious?

Can you forgo making infused butter or oil and simply stir ground bud into your foods? Sure you can, but more often than not you shouldn't because the flavor and textural quality of the finished product will suffer. That said, there are a few exceptions when cooking with dried cannabis flowers works well, provided the buds are finely ground. Meatballs, meat loaves, and other ground meat mixtures, especially those containing lots of other seasonings and ingredients, make good vehicles to carry ground bud. You can also get away with adding it as you would any other herb near the end of cooking, in strongly flavored sauces such as Italian-style tomato sauces or Mexican-style cooked chile salsas.

COOKING WITH CONCENTRATES

Cooking with concentrates expands the horizon of recipes that can be converted to cannabis cooking. These recipes tend to contain far less fat than the ones that depend on butter or oil to carry the medication, an important consideration for those trying to curb calories or limit fats. Of course, cannabis metabolizes better with some fat; but when you cook with concentrates, you eliminate the need to add extra oil or butter to achieve a proper dose.

When cooking for my own personal use, as opposed to developing recipes for others, I almost always use decarboxylated kief (see Chapter 3). It blends easily into most any

food and has a far milder flavor than typically contained in marijuana-infused butter and oil. As hash and kief contain cannabinoids without much plant material, in practical terms this always means far less herbal flavor in the finished food.

Hash and kief can be used interchangeably in recipes, although because heat activates the cannabis, avoid using kief in uncooked recipes unless you decarboxylate it first. Specific dosing ranges can be found in this chapter.

As we discussed earlier in this book, kief and hash can range from dry and crumbly to sticky and gummy. Most smokers prefer the latter, but, for cooking purposes, the dry, crumbly, powdery stuff is easiest to work with. Good news—it's usually less expensive too.

Dry hash is easier to grind, which then allows you to stir the fine powder into all kinds of foods, something impossible to do with the gummy type. If you plan on dissolving the hash in a hot liquid, however, either type will work fine. Once dissolved, the kief or hash is easy to incorporate evenly into the food.

In some creamy foods, the concentrates can add a slight gritty texture, just enough to let you know it's there. In other dishes, the hash or kief completely disappears into the texture of the food.

HOW TO:
The Dos and Don'ts of Cooking with Cannabis

Do include some sort of fat in the recipe so the THC can bind to it. If you medicate a fat-free recipe, be sure something with a fat content accompanies it when you eat.

Don't grind your plant material into a fine powder before making butter or oil with it.

Do finely grind hash or kief before adding to recipes. For hard chunks, a microplane works well, or use as fine a grater as you have. A coffee or spice grinder reserved for cannabis use makes quick work of grinding most hash, except the extremely gummy varieties.

Do make sure your recipe is heated when cooking with kief. Hash, along with marijuana-infused butter and oils, has already been heated/decarboxylated, so additional cooking is optional.

Don't heat your edibles too much because THC is rendered useless at 392 degrees F and loss occurs before that. Whenever possible, cook at low temperatures for longer periods of time.

Don't fry or sauté in medicated oil; it will get too hot and render the THC useless.

Don't use medicated oils for marinades. Very little of the oil is absorbed into the food, so most will be discarded.

Do put the cannabis in the food rather than on it. In other words, you'll have better results medicating the part that goes inside a crust or breading than medicating the crust or breading itself.

Do use a heavy hand with spices, extracts, and flavorings—if your original recipe's flavor is too delicate, the herbal flavor of the cannabis will shine through, which is not a good thing for most people.

Don't skip adding water to the mix when making marijuana-infused butter and oils, which allows the fats to infuse at a low, stable temperature.

Do rinse your plant material with a pot of boiling water when straining the butter and oil.

Depending on the recipe, add hash or kief to dishes in these ways:

- If your recipe involves any heated liquids, dissolve the hash or kief in the liquid before proceeding.

- When adding to long-cooking liquids, such as soups and stews, dissolve the concentrate in the liquid about 5 minutes before serving.

- Beat finely grated kief or hash into fat-containing ingredients before incorporating them into the recipe. This works well for foods like mayonnaise, sour cream, cream cheese, yogurt, butter, oil, milk, or beaten eggs.

- Substitute hash or kief for bud or plant material when making cannabis-infused butters or oils. Quick and easy, no muss, no fuss.

COOKING WITH TINCTURES

Tinctures are cannabis concentrates designed to be taken sublingually (under the tongue) and made by steeping marijuana in alcohol or glycerin. When ingested this way, marijuana takes effect almost as quickly as smoking.

I haven't included tincture recipes because there is no need. Just add a few drops—whatever dose you would normally use—to the food you're eating.

I CAN'T BELIEVE I ATE THE WHOLE THING

Getting too strong a dose is a common problem, especially with people who don't have a lot (or any) experience with edible marijuana. In fact, there is no easier way to take too much marijuana than by eating it, and there's no quicker way to get turned off to edibles forever than by ingesting too much cannabis.

Because it can take an hour and a half or more for the medicine to take effect (two to three hours if you didn't take it on an empty stomach), some people think it's not working. And so they eat more. By the time it all kicks in, they realize they've overdone it.

If this happens to you or someone you know, first and foremost, do not panic! It is impossible to ingest a toxic dose of marijuana. Don't take my word for it. Here's what the World Health Organization had to say on the subject: "There are no recorded cases of overdose fatalities attributed to cannabis, and the estimated lethal dose for humans extrapolated from animal studies is so high that it cannot be achieved by users."

In other words, overdosing on marijuana will not kill you. It just does not work that way in the body. It does not slow your respiratory system or cause organ failure, even in extreme doses. So calm down. You don't need to worry about those things.

That said, it is definitely possible to ingest more marijuana than you need or want. When this happens, you may have feelings of uneasiness, anxiety, or even paranoia. You might also feel dizzy, groggy, or nauseated or get chills. Your coordination might be affected, and likewise you may have trouble talking clearly and could lose your balance

HOW TO:

Short Order—Almost Instant Medicated Foods

Short on time? Use these quick and easy medicated food ideas:

- Dress a salad with vinegar and marijuana-infused oil.

- Drizzle medicated olive oil on steamed veggies, fish, or chicken.

- Drizzle medicated oil on the bread of a sub sandwich (you can even do this with store-bought sandwiches).

- Make toasted garlic bread with medicated butter and/or oil.

- Melt a pat of medicated butter on top of grilled meats.

- Melt a pat of medicated butter on pancakes or French toast.

- Stir powdered hash into hot coffee, hot milk tea, or hot chocolate.

- Sprinkle powdered hash over the cheese in a quesadilla or a grilled cheese sandwich.

- Stir powdered hash into chicken, tuna, or egg salad.

- Sprinkle powdered hash over the fillings in an omelet before folding.

- Add powdered hash to smoothie or milkshake ingredients and blend.

when walking. Some people experience heart rate acceleration, which can further increase anxiety.

It goes without saying you should not be driving or operating heavy machinery. The most common real danger in overmedicating comes in the form of falls or accidents related to impairment of motor skills. Likewise, you should especially exercise caution and consult your cannabis physician if you have a medical condition that already causes any of the symptoms listed above. You wouldn't want to dismiss serious signals your body is sending because you attributed them to overmedicating on marijuana.

The best remedy for ingesting too much cannabis is to simply sleep it off. The peak of the effects should take place about an hour after you begin to notice them and then dissipate after that. It's common to feel anxious or hyperactive in the first hour, before becoming tired afterward. Lie down and go to sleep, and, when you wake up a few hours later, it will all be over. Unlike indulging in too much alcohol, you won't even have to deal with a hangover.

Should you discover a given batch of any recipe is stronger than you want it to be, don't discard it! The remedy is simple: consume a smaller portion in order to decrease the dosage.

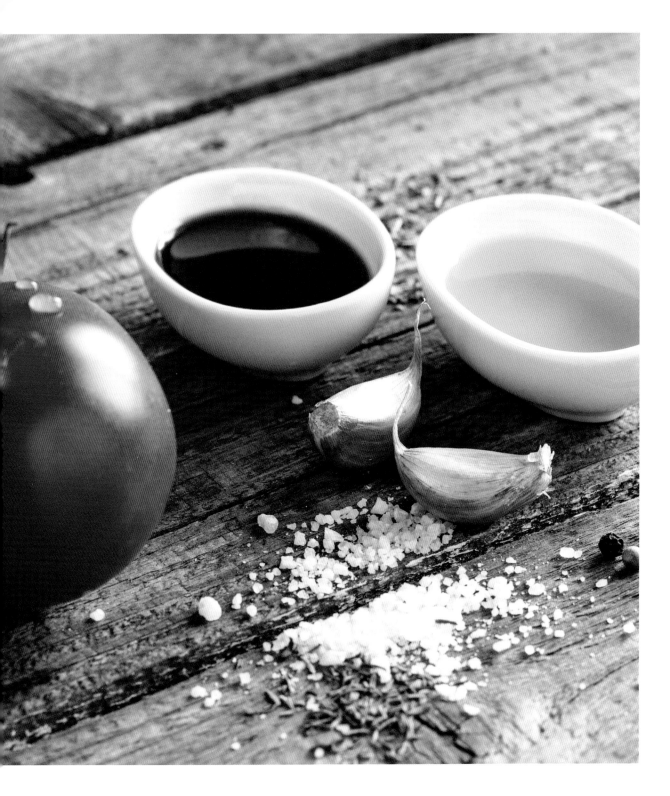

MORE MARIJUANA RECIPES

Enjoy these easy recipes, and, for more, check my website!

Cannaigrette Dressing

This classic "leaded" balsamic vinaigrette is a handy medicated staple to have in your fridge. Besides using it to dress all kinds of fresh salads, trying sprinkling it on steamed veggies or simple grilled chicken or fish.

Suggested serving size: 2 tablespoons
Makes: 6 servings

¼ teaspoon minced garlic
3 tablespoons balsamic vinegar
1 tablespoon water
½ teaspoon Italian seasoning
½ teaspoon black pepper
½ teaspoon salt
6 tablespoons cannabis-infused olive oil
2 tablespoons olive oil

Place all ingredients in a shaker bottle and shake to combine. It will keep in the refrigerator for up to 4 days.

"Baked" Macaroni and Cheese

Here's the quintessential comfort food—creamy, cheesy, and topped with crunchy toasted breadcrumbs.

Makes: 4 servings

3 tablespoons salt
8 ounces elbow macaroni
4 tablespoons cannabutter, divided
2 tablespoons all-purpose flour
1½ teaspoons dry mustard powder
2 cups whole milk
1 small onion, peeled and minced
1 bay leaf
½ teaspoon paprika
2 ounces cream cheese
2½ cups shredded extra-sharp cheddar cheese
½ cup panko breadcrumbs

Preheat oven to 375 degrees F. Spray an 8-inch square baking dish with cooking spray. Add salt to a large stock pot of water and bring to a boil over high heat. Add macaroni and cook until flexible but still al dente. Drain. Melt 2 tablespoons cannabutter in a large saucepan over medium heat. Whisk in flour and mustard powder and cook for 1 minute, whisking constantly. Gradually whisk in milk. Stir in onion, bay leaf, and paprika. Increase heat to bring mixture to a boil. Lower heat to a gentle simmer and cook, stirring frequently, for 15 minutes. Remove from heat and remove bay leaf. Stir in cream cheese and half of the shredded cheddar. Stir until cheese is melted. Season to taste with salt and pepper and stir in prepared macaroni. Spread half the macaroni mixture in the prepared baking pan and sprinkle half the remaining cheese on top of the macaroni. Top with remaining pasta followed by a sprinkling of the remaining cheese.

In a small skillet over medium-low heat, melt remaining 2 tablespoons cannabutter. Toss in panko breadcrumbs and stir to coat. Sprinkle buttered breadcrumbs over the top of the baking dish. Bake for 30 minutes, or until the pasta is bubbling and brown on top.

Dank Chocolate Espresso Brownies

Of course you can make all kinds of foods with cannabis. Nonetheless, the general public still has the perception that "pot brownies" are the thing to have. No matter how big your cannabis cooking repertoire grows, trust me, people are still going to ask for brownies. Give the people what they want. Here is a deep dark dense fudge-like brownie whose flavor is made all the richer by the addition of coffee. This recipe will make a lightly dosed edible. Heavyweights can add some finely ground hash or kief to the batter for extra fortification.

Suggested serving size: 1 brownie
Makes: 9 brownies

½ cup cocoa
½ teaspoon salt
6 tablespoons cannabis-infused butter
6 ounces high-quality dark chocolate
¾ cup all-purpose flour
2 large eggs
2 teaspoons vanilla extract
⅓ cup espresso or strong coffee, cooled
1½ cups sugar
¾ cup chopped walnuts or pecans, optional

Preheat oven to 375 degrees F. Butter an 8-inch square pan and line the bottom and two sides with foil with a little foil hanging over (this will help you lift the brownies out of the pan later). Lightly butter the foil and set aside.

Combine flour, cocoa, and salt (and extra hash or kief if using) and stir to combine. Set aside.

In a small saucepan, melt butter with chocolate over medium-low heat. Set aside to cool slightly.

Whisk eggs, vanilla, and espresso together. Whisk in sugar, followed by melted chocolate mixture. Use a large spoon or rubber spatula to stir in dry ingredients. Stir in nuts, if using. Pour batter into prepared pan using rubber spatula to make a smooth even layer. Bake for about 25 minutes—brownies will be slightly soft in the center. Cool completely in the pan before using the foil to gently lift out and cut into portions. Chill first for easier cutting.

Freezer-friendly: Wrap extra portions in plastic wrap and then foil, label, and freeze for longer storage. Just thaw and enjoy.

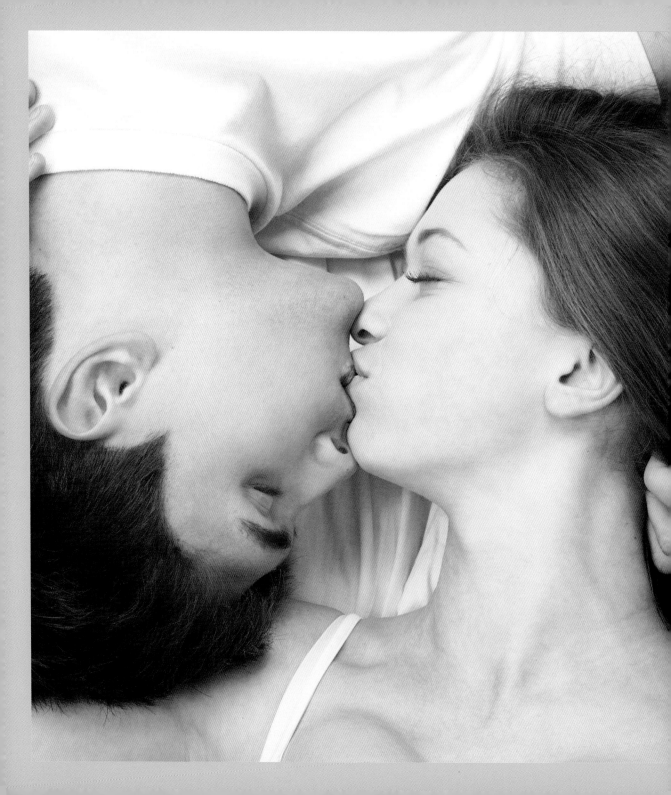

CHAPTER 10

the CANNA SUTRA: BUDS in the BEDROOM

Marijuana and sex! Let's get right to it, ladies: Does weed make sex better?

For most people, the answer is yes. Some studies suggest about two-thirds of users get off on the marijuana-sex combo meal, but judging from the amount of erotica and porn that starts with the participants smoking marijuana, I'm guessing the actual statistic is, *ahem*, "higher."

For me, personally, the answer is a resounding yes! But then it also improves washing dishes, taking out the trash, doing the laundry, and walking the dog on a rainy night. So it goes without saying that it can take sex, which was really damn good to begin with, to new highs. (Pun intended!)

Mary Jane's reputation as an aphrodisiac is deeply ingrained for good reason—it has some real physiological effects. In fact, being high and being sexually aroused have a lot in common, as both affect the brain and hormonal systems. Cannabinoids even have a molecular structure similar to some hormones and can replicate some of their effects.

While there is no scientific evidence that cannabis works like Viagra, marijuana does dilate blood vessels and increase blood flow. (Ancient Indian tantric practitioners were said to use it for that very reason. See the recipe for Bhang Lassi at the end of this chapter for more information!) Besides the obvious performance advantage of increased blood flow during sex for men, it also can heighten sensations for women, so you and your lover might find Mary Jane makes your lovemaking more sensuous and the pleasure of physical touch a bit more intense. It can even make orgasm easier to achieve.

Cannabis can also increase relaxation, and with that comes lower inhibitions. If you or your lover are feeling stressed out, try a nice indica or indica-dominant hybrid. If your love life has lost a little luster and you need a little nudge to try something new or creative, try a good sativa or sativa hybrid to bring energy and spark back.

In and of itself, the act of sharing a joint, pipe, or vaporizer while staring into your lover's eyes in anticipation of what comes next creates a certain level of sensuous intimacy that has primal roots in ancient cannabis fertility rituals. With some lovers, this sharing of cannabis becomes an integral part of the experience.

But it needn't be that serious.

Cannabis combined with sex means different things to different couples, from a novel way to add some sizzle to a lackluster sex life to a natural part of foreplay (and sometimes after-play—far healthier than a post-coitus cigarette) to a spiritual experience. It can be a deeply moving and sensuous experience that opens both parties to trust and intimacy. Or it can be a playful interlude before some hot fun in the sack that leaves you both giggling uncontrollably. It can even be both—depending on the time, place, and mood of the participants.

TIPS FOR TAKING MARY JANE TO BED

Here are some dos and don'ts for making Mary Jane a safe and pleasurable part of your sex life.

- Don't arrive at your rendezvous empty-handed. Do take a hint from singer-songwriter Ashley Monroe (see Chapter 13) and bring "Weed Instead of Roses."

- Do take another lead from Ashley and include a few accouterments. She mentions whips and chains, which is great if you are into such things. Other options might include a blindfold, feathers, whipped cream, handcuffs (or a scarf), or any number of sex toys. Let Mary Jane be the metaphorical libidinous lubricant to more adventurous sex, whatever that means to you.

- Do enjoy a slow, relaxing, sensuous massage with cannabis lotion or hemp oil. Trading massages is a great way to create intimacy and turn your lover on most anytime, but, when Mary Jane is in the room with you, it can help take your sex life to new heights. No, it won't make you or your partner high, but, since cannabinoids can be absorbed through the skin, a massage with either a marijuana-infused oil that you make yourself (see Chapter 9) or one of the commercial cannabis topicals on the market (see Chapter 7) can provide extra relaxation and pain relief, as well as intensify pleasurable sensations. What's not to like?

- Do use caution when smoking in bed; after all, you are still smoking in bed and, even if you are not sleeping, there's lots going on to distract you.

- Do use a bag-style vaporizer that gives you the convenience of inflating the bag once and taking a hit anytime you want it—no waiting for the vape to heat up. Alternately, a portable pen-style vape can remain always at the ready.

- Don't use your bong in the bedroom—nothing can ruin a romantic mood quicker than stinky bong water spilled on the sheets.

- Generally, don't rely on edibles. Not only does edible marijuana cause worse cottonmouth than smoked or vaped cannabis, but the dosing can be too unpredictable. You might be raring to go while your partner is passed out asleep, or vice versa. They also take an hour or more to take effect. However, if you and your partner are experienced with marijuana edibles, the Bhang Lassi recipe in this chapter does make a nice exotic spiced cannabis-laced beverage to share.

SMOKING SHOTGUN-STYLE

One of today's most sensuous smoking practices actually has its origins in war. The practice of *shotgunning a hit* originates with Vietnam War soldiers who turned their weapons into pipes—stoners can create a pipe out of nearly anything. After fitting the chamber with a loaded, lit bowl of cannabis, one buddy would blow smoke down the barrel of the shotgun to his friend who was inhaling at the business end.

Decades later, people *shotgun* without any weaponry involved. For a simple, sensuous "shotgun light" version, one person takes a big hit from a pipe or joint and blows the smoke into her partner's mouth. Experienced stoners will complain this is not truly shotgunning. Maybe not, but it is easy, safe, and sexy and involves no risk of burned lips or ash on the tongue.

That said, with a little care, actually shotgun smoking a joint can bring you and your partner closer together—physically and emotionally. To do it, you take the lit joint in your mouth, and the unlit end is positioned a fraction of an inch from your partner's mouth. You blow, while your partner sucks. Expect a turbo-charged hit, bigger and more potent than average. Shotgun etiquette is a little like oral sex etiquette—be sure to switch positions so your partner gets a turn too!

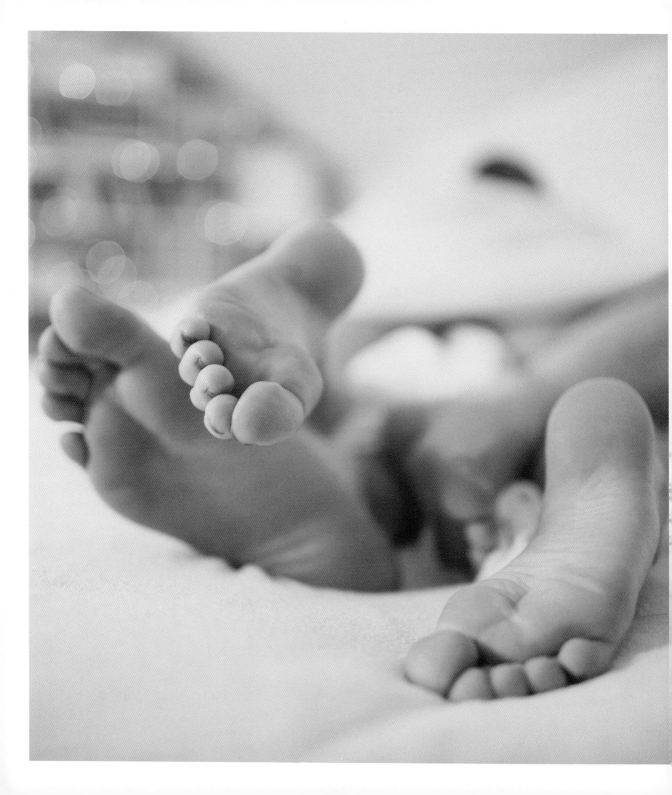

Needless to say, if you aren't careful, things can go wrong. Blistered lips will not enhance your experience. If you decide to try shotgunning, put these tips into practice.

- When it comes to taking the hit, do it quickly as the mouth of the person holding the lit end will get hot fast!

- Take a drink of water and have plenty of saliva present to keep your mouth moist if you have the lit end.

- Use a reasonably long joint so you can keep the burning part well away from your lips.

- Tap off as much ash as possible before beginning.

- Position the burning end in the center of your mouth, away from your tongue or the insides of your cheeks.

OVERCOMING COTTON MOUTH

Xerostomia, or dry mouth (cotton mouth, in stoner terms), is the most common side effect of ingesting marijuana. Most of the time this presents nothing more than a minor inconvenience, but, in regard to sex, when you will be putting your mouth, lips, and tongue to good use, it can interfere with proper technique. Here are some tips to mitigate it.

- Always have a glass of ice water nearby for a quick sip, and try to drink a lot of water ahead of time so you're not dehydrated.

- If wine or other alcoholic drinks, and even coffee, are part of the night's festivities, know that these drinks are all diuretics that can exacerbate the problem of dry mouth.

- Eat something with a little cayenne pepper or suck on hard candies, both of which stimulate saliva production.

- Store-bought mouthwash contains alcohol. Try an herbal remedy instead: Pour 1 teaspoon dried rosemary, 1 teaspoon dried mint, and 1 teaspoon dried aniseed into 2½ cups boiling water and steep for 20 minutes. Strain out the herbs and refrigerate. Use as an all-natural germ-fighting, breath-freshening, nondehydrating gargle.

BUZZ KILLER: CANNABIS COITUS IS NOT FOR EVERYONE

According to studies, not everyone finds that marijuana enhances sex. *Psychology Today* cites several small studies with mixed results—roughly a third of people said marijuana did not enhance their sexual experiences, a finding the magazine says is "pharmacologically unique" because the sexual effects of other mood-altering drugs are fairly consistent.

Marijuana's sexual effects cover the spectrum from inhibiting to enhancing. For instance, some studies indicate that marijuana can help erectile function, but at least one shows it might exacerbate erectile dysfunction. In my own personal research, I have yet to encounter a stoner guy with issues. Drinkers, well, they're another story.

You may ask yourself, Why, if marijuana's physiological effects are already documented, can the effect of cannabis on sex be so varied? Several factors might be at play.

- The strain may not be right for that person. As we discussed in Chapter 1, some sativa strains make some people anxious and paranoid, and some indica strains induce couch-lock. Either extreme can kill passion.

- The dosage may be off. Dosing with marijuana is never a one-size-fits-all situation. What may be right for one partner may be too much for another.

- Marijuana is not a sex therapist or miracle cure. While it can help lower inhibitions and heighten pleasure, sexual hang-ups or dysfunctions will not simply disappear.

- Marijuana can make you hyper-aware, which can be good or bad. If there are problems in your relationship, pot can highlight rather than reduce them.

HOW TO:

Making Bhang Lassi

While the origins of *Bhang Lassi*, a spice- and cannabis-laced drink made with milk or yogurt, remain buried in history, it is said that ancient tantric practitioners used it as an aphrodisiac and to prolong erections. Hmmm, maybe the ancients were on to something.

If you or your partner are cannabis newbies or "lightweights," I don't recommend mixing cannabis edibles and sex (see the dos and don'ts under "Tips for Taking Mary Jane to Bed," pages 118–119). But if you are experienced users who know what dosage of edibles you can handle, give this ancient recipe a try.

There are as many variations on this drink as there are curry blends or marijuana strains. The ingredients in this simple but traditional version shouldn't prove too difficult for most western cooks to find. You can get rosewater at Indian or Middle Eastern grocery stores or gourmet shops. It adds a nice exotic flavor to the drink, but it isn't essential, so don't let lack of rosewater keep you from giving this ancient beverage a try.

MAKES 2 SERVINGS

- 1 cup water
- ½ ounce marijuana (leaves and flowers)
- 2 cups warm milk (or almond milk for a vegan version)
- 1 tablespoon blanched, chopped almonds
- $\frac{1}{16}$ teaspoon garam masala (a mixture of cloves, cinnamon, and cardamom)
- ⅛ teaspoon powdered ginger
- ¼ to ½ teaspoon rosewater
- ½ cup sugar

Bring the water to a rapid boil. If necessary, remove seeds or stem pieces from the marijuana and add to the boiling water. Turn off the heat and let the mixture steep for about 10 minutes. Strain through a small strainer or a piece of cheesecloth, squeezing as much water as possible from the marijuana. Set the infused water aside.

Place the wet cannabis in a mortar and add 2 tablespoons of warm milk. Firmly grind the leaves into the milk. Gather up the marijuana, place in the strainer or cheesecloth and squeeze out as much milk as you can, and put it in a small bowl. Repeat this process until you have about ¼ cup of milk. By this point the cannabis will have turned into a pulpy mass. Add the chopped almonds to it along with more warm milk. Grind this into a fine paste. Squeeze the paste to collect the extract as before. Repeat until the milk is gone and all that is left are some fibers and nut meal, which can be discarded.

Add the garam masala, powdered ginger, rosewater, and sugar to the milk. Stir in the infused water. Serve warm, chilled, or over ice.

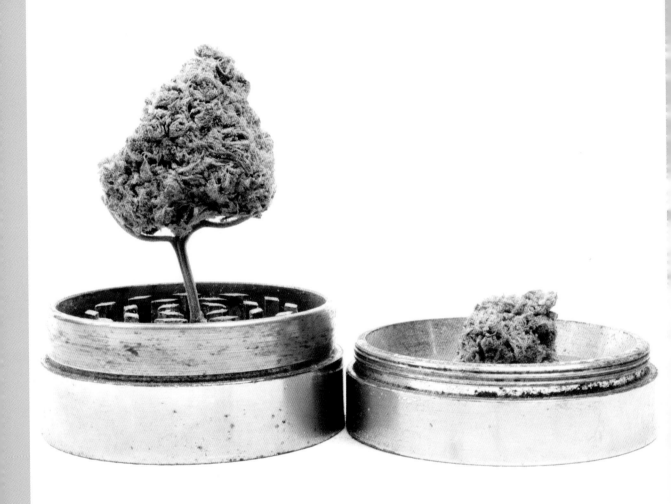

CHAPTER 11
MARIJUANA MAMAS: CANNABIS *and* PARENTING

The topic of mothers using marijuana is one that elicits a knee-jerk reaction of horror from the uninformed. Yet these same people tend to think nothing of women who regularly indulge in a glass of wine or a cocktail in front of their children

Once again, it's all about stigma and misinformation. The truth is, many parents claim their marijuana use actually improves their parenting abilities! Sometimes it's because cannabis can help with medical and health issues more effectively and with fewer side effects than traditional pharmaceuticals. More often than not, though, it's because marijuana helps to keep these busy mothers more relaxed, patient, and focused, and better able to enjoy simple parent-child bonding experiences.

Diane Fornbacher, executive editor of *Ladybud* magazine and a cannabis activist, says people often jump to the wrong conclusion when they hear women saying marijuana makes them better parents. Diane says it has nothing whatsoever to do with the ability to parent, but rather it encourages a dynamic that helps parents relate to their kids.

"I never use cannabis to cope with my children, and in fact, I spend much more time around my children *without* ingesting cannabis than I do after consuming it," says Diane. "We read together, play in the park, hunt for minerals in the Rocky Mountains, use miniature construction equipment in the sandbox and ride bikes together. I have also been around my children after I have consumed cannabis legally. It didn't affect my interactions with them adversely—in fact, it didn't change how I felt about them or the way I treated them, just as they felt no differently toward me. However," she adds, "it did make Play-Doh, coloring books and

Legos far more interesting to me, which in turn made it easier to bond with my kids over these things."

CANNABIS CONVERSATIONS

Talking about marijuana is a tough subject for a lot of parents, whether it be their own use or their child's potential use. Our nation's diverse marijuana laws only complicate it further. I am not a parent, but I spoke with many parents for this book, most of whom are involved in the cannabis movement and have a lot of experience with the subject, as well as the public's reactions to it. With few exceptions, the parents I spoke with believed honesty was the best policy—albeit at the right time and in the proper context.

When parents choose to have The Talk about marijuana use with their children usually falls into two age ranges: younger kids, usually still in elementary school, and teenagers. Many parents like to wait until the junior high and high school years, when they know their kids will likely be exposed to marijuana from outside sources. Parents usually prefer that their children learn the truth about the effects and risks of pot use at home, instead of hearing hyped-up propaganda from school authorities or misinformation from their friends.

Other parents prefer to talk to their kids about marijuana earlier, when their children are in elementary school. Sometimes it's a school unit on drugs or a presentation from DARE that raises the topic—and for some parents, like Deanna, a thirty-nine-year-old Minnesota mother of four, medical issues forced the talk. Deanna sat her kids down after being reunited with them following a brain surgery.

"We talked openly and honestly, and they watched me trade out my medications from the pharmacy with natural medicine," she says. "I don't medicate in front of my kids, I never have, but I know they have talked to their friends about it and educated them about it."

Oregon mom Lindsey, who uses cannabis to treat her multiple sclerosis, says she just got tired of hiding it, so she stopped. She talked to her kids in an age-appropriate manner about what marijuana is—and isn't—and how it helped her. She also explained that they lived in a state where using marijuana to treat disease was illegal, which is why she had to keep her medicine a secret. Now her family has moved to Oregon, and she can finally have safe, legal access to the plant that best treats her serious medical condition. (And I'm happy to report that all fourteen pharmaceutical medications she once needed to survive in an illegal state have been replaced with cannabis. Amazing!)

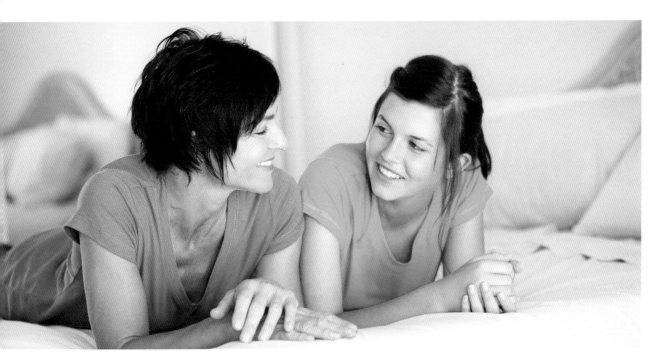

For those who want their children to understand the truth about cannabis, consider these tips.

- Talking to kids about marijuana is a lot like talking to them about sex. Keep it simple and at a level the child can grasp.

- "Marijuana as medicine" is a great way for younger kids to grasp the concept. A first grader can understand that a plant can help with Mommy's migraine, but she's unlikely to grasp the complexities of constitutional law and the political implications of the war on drugs.

- As that first grader gets older, the more complex issues surrounding marijuana can make great teaching vehicles and help to get kids interested in subjects like science, health, civics, government, and more. In fact, the subject is a perfect one for high school research projects and essay themes on the debate over cannabis.

- Turn on the tube! Orange County, California, dad Robert sat his entire family down for a viewing of the documentary, *What If Cannabis Cured Cancer* (see Chapter 13), to begin an honest discussion about marijuana with his three kids. This and other well-researched but easy-to-follow documentaries can provide the perfect place to start a discussion with kids old enough to understand.

- "Do as I say, not as I do": Without a doubt, one of the biggest dilemmas facing parents is how to discourage their kids from using marijuana without seeming hypocritical. The parents I talked to again cited honesty. They explained to their teen and tween kids that there are substances like marijuana and alcohol that are for adult use only. They also took time to explain there isn't enough research on marijuana and the developing brain to know what kind of damage marijuana can cause in young people. The ultimate message should be: *Wait until you are an adult to decide whether or not to use marijuana.*

MEDICAL MARIJUANA FOR CHILDREN

The Internet is filled with tragic stories of children fighting devastating and often fatal diseases who have suddenly been given a ray of hope in the form of medical cannabis. CNN's chief medical correspondent, Dr. Sanjay Gupta, had an epiphany and reversed his prior anti-marijuana stance largely because he met Charlotte Figi. Young Charlotte suffered from more than 300 grand mal seizures a week, and her parents, who had tried every remedy available, were at their wit's end. Now with cannabis therapy, Charlotte's seizures occur only two or three times per month.

When politicians talk about marijuana for children, those that do agree tend to do so reluctantly, as a last-ditch effort when absolutely everything else has failed. But why should this be? Cannabis is one of the safest therapeutic substances in existence, with no serious side effects. Shouldn't it be the first substance tried before exposing children to a host of toxic chemicals that come with a cornucopia of serious side effects?

That was the philosophy of Erin Purchase and husband Brandon Krenzler, who began treating their daughter Mykayla with cannabinoid therapy even before treating her with pharmaceuticals. Just after her seventh birthday, Mykayla was diagnosed with intermediate risk T-cell acute lymphoblastic leukemia that had metastasized to her brain and spinal fluid.

"Many parents and physicians think of cannabinoid therapy as a last resort option when treating their child's illness. I believe that beginning Mykayla's cannabis therapy from the very start has played a major role in keeping her body strong through fighting

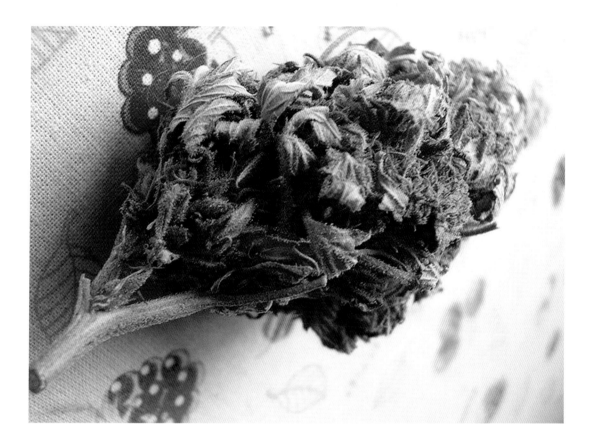

cancer and chemotherapy without any pharmaceutical based symptom relievers, such as narcotic painkillers," says Erin.

The couple decided to try cannabis therapy because they had already witnessed its medicinal benefits firsthand while treating Erin's severe metabolic condition. They began administering cannabis oil to Mykayla ten days post-diagnosis. Her parents say Mykayla did not spend a single day in pain, she did not lose a single pound, and if it were not for the

chemo causing her hair to fall out, you would not have known she even had cancer.

The results cemented Erin and Brandon's resolve to do everything in their power to help others facing similar circumstances. Purchase says, "I witnessed my little girl go from the sickest she has ever been to a smiling happy child with no cancer in her body. Seeing this firsthand gave me the motivation to step up my activism and spread our story as far as I could get it. No child should have

SAFETY PATROL:

Advice on Kids and Cannabis from a CPS Attorney

Jen Ani, an attorney based in San Rafael, California, and specializing in helping parents with Child Protective Services issues, has handled many cases that involved marijuana use in a home where children live. Ani says there are important steps parents can take to keep their families safe from persecution over one or more parent's responsible cannabis use.

The first thing Ani stressed is the importance of where you live. If you live in a legal or medically legal state, you're offered protection against legal persecution like having your children placed into foster care or you being found an unfit parent, which can result in the children being placed up for adoption. However, if you live in a state where marijuana remains illegal on all levels, the authorities can take your children from you if they find marijuana in your home.

Geography still comes into play in legal states. For instance, in Marin County, California, where Ani lives, Child Protective Services has no problem with either recreational or medicinal use of marijuana, providing there are no other legal or safety issues. However, some individual counties practice zero tolerance for parents using medical marijuana, despite the fact that it has been legal in California for more than seventeen years.

Keep in mind too that legal problems don't only involve Child Protective Services or the police. Justified or not, a parent's marijuana use is often used as a weapon in custody battles.

Ultimately, Ani says, the number one reason kids are removed from a home is a general "failure to protect" or "failure to supervise." You must be sure your drug use—whether it be cannabis, doctor-prescribed pharmaceuticals, or anything else—does not have an adverse effect on your child. Ani also cautions that, though it is unfair, single parents are typically judged more harshly.

Here are her words of wisdom on proactively protecting your family in case you ever run into a legal issue concerning parenting and cannabis use:

- Establish good relationships with your pediatrician, children's teachers, day care workers, and other caregivers. This is important in case you ever need to call on them to vouch for your level of responsibility and regular care for your children.

- In general, don't be a flake. If you are, or are even perceived as one, regardless of the reasons, your marijuana use will likely take the brunt of the legal blame.

- Always present well. Make sure your child arrives for school in clean clothes and well fed. Every time a kid has missed breakfast or says "I'm hungry" at school can turn into a potential problem. Your cannabis use can get blamed for you not regularly caring for your child.

to suffer if there is something like cannabis oil available to help them. Far too many children lay sick in hospital beds for weeks on end in excruciating pain, feeding tubes in their noses and a sad look about their faces. This is not the case in the majority of children treated with cannabis. Until this is an option for every parent throughout the world, our job as activists is not done and I will continue to spread the truth about this amazing plant."

Her child's illness also inspired Dr. Lakisha Jenkins to get more involved with cannabis therapy, although it was too late to treat her own daughter, Kiona, who suffered from a rare type of brain tumor that had no specific treatment protocol. Even though Jenkins holds a doctorate in naturopathy, is registered as a professional herbalist with the American Herbalist Guild, and has a bachelor of science degree in holistic nutrition, she was prevented from using alternative therapies on her daughter. Medical social workers and Child Protective Services informed Jenkins that, because Kiona was a minor, Jenkins could not offer her cannabis therapies.

"The State of California has the ability to intervene when a parent wants to do anything against conventional medical advice," explains Jenkins. Kiona did defeat her brain tumor, but by that time the effects of chemotherapy and radiation had taken their toll. She passed away just twelve days shy of her twelfth birthday.

In her practice, Dr. Lakisha Jenkins treats patients, both children and adults, with cannabis and other healing herbs, blended in specific formulas for the individual patients' conditions and needs. "Herbs are actual nutrition and are metabolized by our bodies," she says. "When you introduce herbal plant extracts in whole plant form, including but not limited to cannabis, it allows your body to get the full benefit of and interact with the constituents of that plant and utilize the portions that are beneficial and discard the rest. In general, herbs are safe and effective. Negative side effects are only a consideration if there is an identified allergy to a specific botanical and/or the compounds found within or if there is a possibility for negative interaction with pharmaceuticals."

When asked what advice she'd give to parents who are considering alternative therapies for their children, Jenkins says, "Research, research, research! Especially in the case of children, you as a parent are charged with being their health advocate. Just as no one can tell you as an individual how your body works better than you, no one knows your child better than you do. There are options, both natural and conventional. Be sure that you are secure in knowing that the treatment options that you choose are the best that are available for your child and your situation."

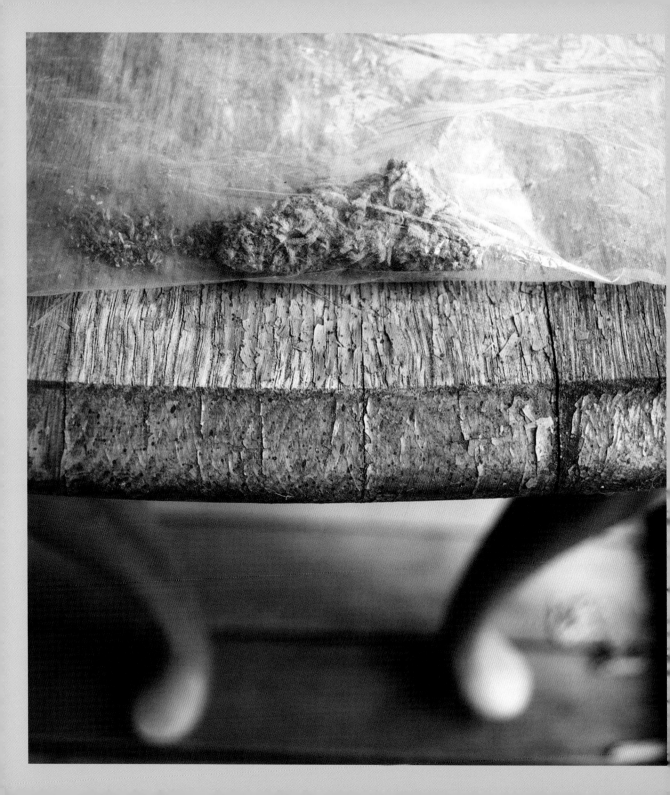

CHAPTER 12

HANDY HEMPY HOUSEHOLD HINTS: POT PARTIES, DIY PROJECTS, KEEPING *your* GREEN CLEAN, *and* MORE

Most women's magazines and helpful hints columns distinctly lack marijuana content. Until the time comes when we open up an issue of *Woman's Day* and see helpful hints for hosting a tasting party, cleaning your bong, navigating stoner etiquette dilemmas, crafting with cannabis, and finding thrifty ways to improve your marijuana experience, I will try to fill in the gaps!

ENTERTAINING: HOST A PRIVATE MARIJUANA-TASTING PARTY!

"Cannabis Cuisine Goes Gourmet" news stories in hip urban publications have been peppered with reports of secret underground dinner parties. At these parties, talented chefs not only medicate their food but match specific marijuana strains to specific foods for the pure culinary appeal of creating haute cuisine in which the flavor of the marijuana enhances the finished product, as opposed to being a detracting necessary evil.

If you're not lucky enough to score an invitation to one of these soirees, think about hosting your own. When you mix a group of your best buds with some great foods, how could everyone not have a good time?

Marijuana-Tasting Party Tips

- If you are doing a tasting party and you plan to medicate every course, use a light hand when it comes to dosing. A VERY light hand. Unless otherwise noted, marijuana recipes are written with the assumption that you will be

POT PARTY MIX

Be careful to portion out this party mix. I purposely dosed it lightly because it's easy to keep on snacking and overdo it. Depending on what you have on hand or your dietary requirements, you can use cannabis-infused butter or olive oil for this recipe. If you want a stronger dose, stir some decarboxylated kief (see Chapter 3) or finely grated hash into the mix to fortify it.

MAKES: 6 CUPS

SUGGESTED SERVING SIZE: 1 CUP

- 3 cups Chex cereal, corn, rice, wheat, or mix and match more than one
- 1 cup bite-size cheddar crackers
- 1 cup thin pretzel sticks
- 1 cup roasted peanuts
- ¼ cup cannabis-infused butter (melted) or olive oil (at room temperature)
- 2 tablespoons Worcestershire sauce
- 1 teaspoon seasoned salt
- ¾ teaspoon garlic powder
- ¾ teaspoon onion powder
- ⅛ teaspoon cayenne pepper, more to taste, optional

Preheat oven to 250 degrees F. Combine cereal, crackers, pretzels, and peanuts in a large bowl and stir to mix. Spread on a large baking sheet.

If using butter, melt on the stove top over low heat or in the microwave. Combine melted cannabis butter or oil with Worcestershire sauce, seasoned salt, garlic powder, onion powder, and cayenne pepper and whisk to mix. Pour over mixture on baking pan and stir to coat the ingredients well. Bake for 50 minutes, stirring every 10 to 15 minutes. Remove from oven and let cool completely. Store in an airtight container or portion into plastic bags and seal.

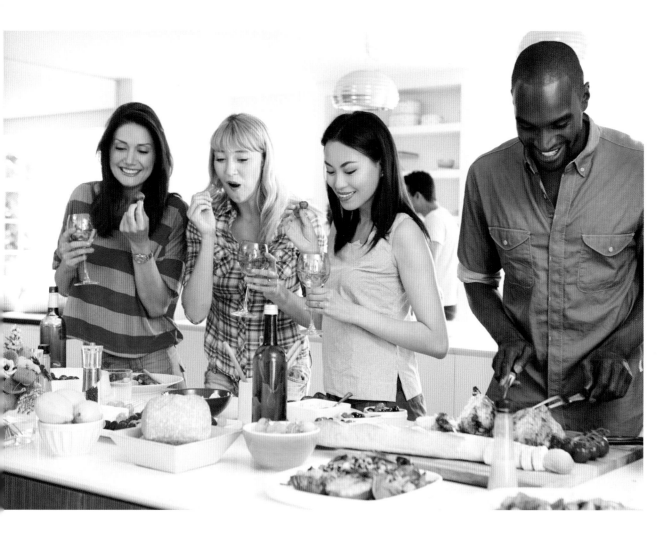

consuming only one medicated food at a time. Plan how many foods you will be serving and reduce the dosage in each accordingly so your guests aren't asleep by the end of the night. It's easier to make better-tasting foods with lower doses, so the flavors of your foods will shine!

- Consider making it a potluck. (Yes, that pun was definitely intended!) Assign each person a different course to bring to the party. Take care to make sure everyone who is contributing knows the rule about using a light dose (see above).

- Consider a theme for your party so you'll end up with a cohesive group of dishes that complement one another. The easiest theme is based on ethnic foods: Italian, Japanese, Greek, Mexican, or any other international cuisine. You can narrow that theme into specific regional specialties too (New Orleans Mardi Gras party, anyone?). Seasonal harvests make great themes that let you cook sustainably. Another fun party plan involves guests bringing lots of different versions of the same dish: think chili cook-off, barbecue competition, soup and salad buffet, or grilled cheese party. I know you'll come up with lots of other themes.

- Keep it discreet. Your marijuana-tasting party is not the kind of event to blast out to your Facebook or Twitter followers. Not only will you be overrun with too many "guests," but you may attract the attention of unwanted guests as well as law enforcement. Major buzzkills all.

- Designate a driver. A lot of people have a low tolerance for edibles. Have a plan in place for those who shouldn't drive and/ or expect to have some overnight guests.

" Of course I know how to roll a joint. "

——*Martha Stewart*

A CLEAN PIPE IS A HAPPY PIPE

The better quality your weed, the quicker your pipes and bongs will get dirty. If you let things go too long, the airways will get clogged up with thick, sticky black resin.

The best way to unclog a pipe in the short term is with a poker. Metal makes the best pokers. For best results, take your lighter and run it up and down the length of the metal poker for a few seconds until it is very hot, and then use it to ream out the pipe. The heat will help to melt the sticky tar-like resins clogging the pipe and make them easier to remove.

No matter how often you ream out your pipes, eventually—and better sooner than later—you will need to clean them. Yes, you can find any number of commercial pipe and bong cleaners on the market. But, no, you do not really need any of them. I have tried many of them, and for my money, none works better than a 92 percent or higher grade isopropyl alcohol, the kind you can buy at just about any drugstore. It's easy to find and inexpensive and

DESIGNER JOINTS AND ROACH PAPER ART

Once you've perfected your joint-rolling skills as outlined in Chapter 2, you may want to step it up a notch and make it more fancy. A quick Internet search will yield detailed step-by-step text and/or video instructions for accomplishing the fancier designs. Here are some ideas to check out.

- Pump up the potency. Try sprinkling some ground hash or kief over the plant material, or adding some cannabis wax or oil to the mix for a super-strong joint.

- Cannabis cones. Cone-shaped joints, sometimes known as Dutch joints, are a popular alternative to traditional cylinders. Some people prefer the way the shape smokes, so give it a try to see if you like it. You can find rolling instructions on the Internet that use ordinary rolling papers, or you can purchase special pre-rolled cone papers that you simply fill and twist closed, making it easy for anyone to make perfect Dutch joints.

- Dutch tulip. The easiest of the sculptural designer joints to roll, this flower-shaped smokable never ceases to impress, both before and after combustion.

- Make it big. Giant, oversized submarine sandwiches are a casual party menu staple. Why not add a huge oversized party joint to the mix next time too? An Internet search for "monster joint rolling" will show you how. Be sure to have plenty of bud on hand—giant joints are hungry monsters that can eat up your stash.

- Stoners are a creative bunch, and a net search for "origami joint rolling" will prove it. You'll find joints that multiple people can smoke at once, along with all manner of sculptural creations whose medium consists of rolling papers and ground ganja.

- Search for "roach paper art images" and be prepared to be blown away. You will never look at the burned-down ends of a marijuana cigarette in the same way again. Michelangelo himself would be amazed. Some of the more enthusiastic joints smokers out there are sitting on veritable art supply warehouses. Go forth and create!

dissolves even the toughest mess. Don't forget that you can clean your pipe screens in alcohol as well; just rinse them well before using.

You can use weaker rubbing alcohols too; just be prepared to scrub a little. Either way, I like to wear rubber or latex gloves when cleaning pipes because the black liquid gets under my nails and never smells good.

The following method works for most pipes and bongs except wooden ones. Immerse small pipes or bong pieces in alcohol and let soak for 15 minutes or more.

Before rinsing, add a little something to the pipe along with the alcohol to break particles loose. To each pipe (aside from one hitters) add a half teaspoon to several tablespoons (depending on pipe or bong size) of coarse rock salt, uncooked rice grains, and/or cracked ice and swirl it all around with the alcohol. Use a pipe cleaner to ream the mixture through tight spaces and tubes. Rinse well and repeat if necessary for sparkling clean glass or metal pipes and bongs that look as new as the day you bought them.

Cleaning Wooden Pipes

Avoid using alcohol—or even water—on wooden pipes. To clean the airways, use a hot metal poker to ream out as much resin as you can. Do this process often, after every two or three smoking sessions, so that you never allow a large amount to build up.

To clean the bowl, you can use a small knife to scrape out buildup or, better yet, crumple up a small ball of aluminum foil and use it to scrub the bowl. Whichever you use, take care never to scrape your wooden pipe down to bare wood; always leave a thin protective coating of black carbon.

In a Pinch: Pipe Pokers Buried in Your Cupboard

A clogged pipe or bong with nary a poker in sight can be a frustrating thing, but chances

THE BUZZ:

BARGAIN VAPORIZER BAGS

If you own a Volcano or other bag-type vaporizer, you can get replacement bags for it anytime at your local grocery store. Turkey bags that allow you to bake the bird in the bag in the oven are made out of the same material as vaporizer bags. Depending on the brand and model you own, you may need to replace the valve in order to use it on a turkey bag, but it's worth it for the lower cost and easy access to vape bags anytime. The turkey bags are often larger than the bags that come with most vapes, a convenient plus, especially if you are entertaining.

are you have something lying around the house that can get the job done. The suitability of the items below will, of course, depend on the size and shape of the pipe or bong piece you are attempting to unclog. But consider using any of the following:

- Heavy duty paper clips—straighten them to form a poker.

- Baked potato nails—found in every 1950s kitchen, the same metal "nails" that helped your baked potatoes cook evenly can also help ream out your pipes.

- Hardware nails—long, thin hardware nails can also do the job.

- Barbecue skewers—depending on the size of the pipe, metal and/or wooden skewers can sometimes clear the passages.

- Knitting needles—you have to knit fine yarns to have a needle thin enough to work as a poker, but they exist.

DIY!

Put a bunch of stoners together with nothing to smoke out of and all of a sudden, one or more people in the group will turn into MacGyver. Pot smokers can turn almost anything into a pipe, a handy skill to have in a pinch or anytime you don't want to travel with paraphernalia. Next time you want to imbibe but you forgot your pipe and don't have any rolling paper, try one of these easy anytime-anywhere solutions and party on!

Totally Tubular

Materials/Tools: Cardboard tube from a roll of toilet paper, aluminum foil, a small knife or other poking implement, and a needle or hairpin.

Directions: Use a small knife (or a key or a pen or a golf tee) to poke a small hole the size of the desired pipe bowl into the cardboard tube about ⅓ of the way from one end. Form the aluminum foil into a small bowl slightly larger than the hole. Very gently, to avoid tearing the foil, poke a few small holes in the bottom of the

bowl using a heavy duty needle, a toothpick, or the end of a paper clip or hairpin. Place the bowl in the hole in the tube, load with ground marijuana, and light the bowl, holding your hand over one end of the tube while inhaling from the other. Remove your hand at the end and inhale all the smoke in the tube.

Smoke Your Vegetables (and Fruits)

Materials/Tools: Ballpoint pen casing, suitable fresh fruits or vegetables. Generally speaking, firmer fruits and veggies like apples, pears, and potatoes make the best pipes, but, if it doesn't have to last long, you can get by with others. I have had some nice flavorful smokes out of cucumbers and even large strawberries.

Directions: We'll use an apple for purposes of illustration as that seems to be the most popular produce pipe, but the principles of how to make it work on lots of different types of produce. One of the best tools to use is the shaft of a cheap plastic ballpoint pen. Remove the ink cartridge and writing tip, insert the pen shaft into the apple about ½-inch from the bottom, and run it through the fruit on the diagonal so that it comes out near the stem on the opposite side. The bottom hole will be used to smoke out of, and the top one will be the carburetor (see Chapter 2). Remove the apple stem and place the pen shaft just next to where it was.

HOW TO:

Crafty, Grafty Marijuana Leaf Chart

Whenever you need to draw a decent marijuana leaf for a crafting project, use this graphed-out design for great results. It's perfect for counted cross-stitch or transferring the design for painting projects. It works for knitting too, but expect a knitted leaf to look like a sativa because of the craft's somewhat elongated stitches.

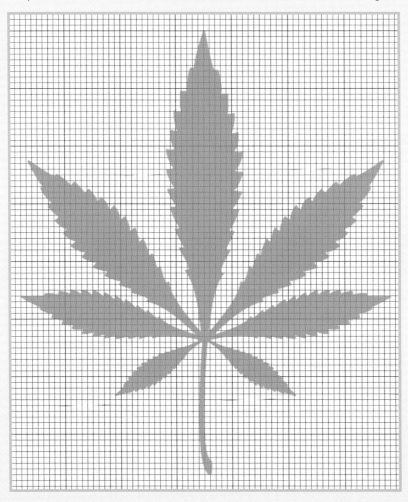

Press the shaft into the apple until it meets up with the first diagonal tunnel you made. Use a knife to carve out a small "bowl" on top where the stem of the apple used to be. You may choose to line the bowl with aluminum foil (as in the tubular pipe or gravity bong) or just add your marijuana directly. Light the cannabis, hold your finger over the carb hole while inhaling from the other, let go of the carb at the last second, and inhale the hit.

Gravity Ganja

Materials/Tools: Empty 2-liter plastic soda or water bottle and cap; another larger bottle, jug, or bucket that can hold the 2-liter bottle—or a sink filled with water; aluminum foil; knife or scissors; and a needle or hairpin.

Directions: Gravity bongs are easy to fashion and they deliver megahits. Start by using the knife or scissors to cut the bottom quarter off the 2-liter bottle. Next, take off the bottle cap and poke about a ½-inch hole in the center of it. Fashion the aluminum foil to fit into the hole in the cap. This will ultimately hold the cannabis. Use a needle, toothpicks, or the end of a hairpin or paper clip to poke four or five small holes in the bottom of the foil. Fill the second, larger container (or sink) about one-half full with water. Screw the cap with the aluminum foil bowl onto the cut, semisubmerged bottle and fill with ground marijuana—be sure

HOW TO:
Storing Your Stash

Proper storage can help keep your marijuana stash fresher and can also help you avoid things like mold. Nobody should smoke moldy weed.

If your marijuana came in a ziplock plastic bag, keep it there in the short term, but that is not the most optimum storage. Airtight glass storage jars work best. You can find jars specifically made for storing marijuana in a variety of sizes, but mason jars or recycled screw-top jars work well too. Get a size that holds everything without having to cram it in and without a lot of extra air space. Too much air can lead to excessive dryness. Store the jars in a cool, dark place.

If your marijuana is not yet fully cured, don't seal it up. Buds should be sticky but not wet because, if moisture is present, mold can grow. If you bought your marijuana from a good dispensary or reputable dealer, this won't be an issue. But if you grow your own or get it from a friend who does, make sure it has had ample time to dry before storing. (See the curing section in Chapter 8.)

to submerge the bottle first, or your weed will fly all over the place!

Ignite the marijuana while slowly pulling the bottle up. This will cause the bottle to fill with smoke. When the bottle is full and just before the bottom is about to clear the water, remove the cap and inhale the smoke.

Voila! You just took your first gravity bong hit.

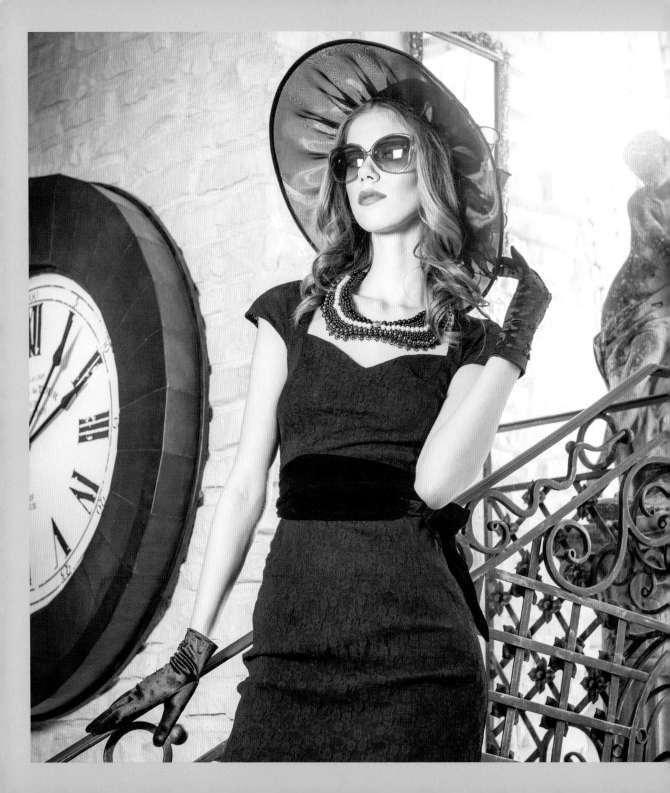

CHAPTER 13

STARRING MARY JANE: CANNABIS *in* ENTERTAINMENT

Movies, music, television, and beyond—Mary Jane is everywhere in pop culture. While it used to be that marijuana was only featured in entertainment for men, the world of weed has opened wide up for women, with female superstars and tastemakers taking the lead on the trail.

HOORAY FOR HOLLYWEED! MARIJUANA IN THE MOVIES

For decades, marijuana has been both celebrated and vilified in film. Early movies like the infamous *Reefer Madness* (1936), and its legion of sensationalistic clones, spoke to the evils of marijuana. They are now viewed as kitschy laughable relics of a bygone era, but in their day they fueled hysteria and helped push forward and cement the prohibitionist agenda.

Fortunately, many of us have evolved to a place where marijuana use is simply seen as a natural everyday part of life, and thankfully its portrayal in some more enlightened movies reflects that. In many cases, just as in real life, it is women, and their use of marijuana, who are the catalysts for pushing the scene and the "normalization" of cannabis use forward.

Paul Mazursky, who passed away in 2014 at the age of eighty-four, began the whole women and weed movie trend back in 1968 in his screenplay of *I Love You, Alice B. Toklas*, in which **Leigh Taylor-Young**'s pot brownies created quite a transformation in Peter Sellers's repressed lawyer character. Even though most early movies kept marijuana use strictly in the domain of men, Mazursky had his female leads, **Natalie Wood** and **Dyan Cannon**, smoking ganja when he wrote and directed *Bob & Ted & Carol & Alice* (1969), a film considered groundbreaking at the time for its exploration of partner swapping and sexual taboos. Later, his acclaimed *An*

Unmarried Woman (1978), included a scene in which a fifteen-year-old girl informed her mother's new boyfriend, "I smoke pot sometimes."

Here are some of the most memorable women with weed on the big screen.

- **Diane Keaton** insists on smoking marijuana before making love with Woody Allen's character in the comedy classic *Annie Hall* (1977). In fact she even tries to convince Allen to join her, saying he might not need therapy if he would only partake.

- **Lily Tomlin**, **Jane Fonda**, and **Dolly Parton** light up while plotting sweet revenge on their abusive boss (Dabney Coleman) in *Nine to Five* (1980). In a later scene, Fonda's character, a cannabis newbie, proudly announces to her ex-husband while asserting her independence: "I smoke pot now!"

- **Susan Sarandon**, a real-life anti–drug war activist, smokes weed both on her own and with her lover (Tim Robbins), in the baseball comedy *Bull Durham* (1988).

- Cannabis is just a regular part of life in *Stealing Beauty* (1996), a visually stunning coming-of-age movie directed by Bernardo Bertolucci that has **Liv Tyler**'s nineteen-year-old character traveling to

> " Rusty thinks I should smoke marijuana, and I did for a while, but it only makes me giggle. What I've found does the most good is just to get into a taxi and go to Tiffany's. "
>
> —*Audrey Hepburn in Breakfast at Tiffany's*

Tuscany after her mother's suicide to discover the identity of her real father and lose her virginity. Some of the film's most memorable scenes include Jeremy Irons as a gay playwright dying of AIDS bonding with Tyler's character over ganja.

- Ten years later and Susan Sarandon is still smoking marijuana on film. This time she costars with **Julia Roberts** in the comedy-drama *Stepmom* (1998), in which Sarandon's character uses medical marijuana to treat her terminal cancer.

- **Cameron Diaz**'s character suggests using Mary Jane as a social stimulant in *Being John Malkovich* (1999). Her strategy works as **Catherine Keener**, the object of desire, ends up rolling a joint for Diaz and her onscreen husband.

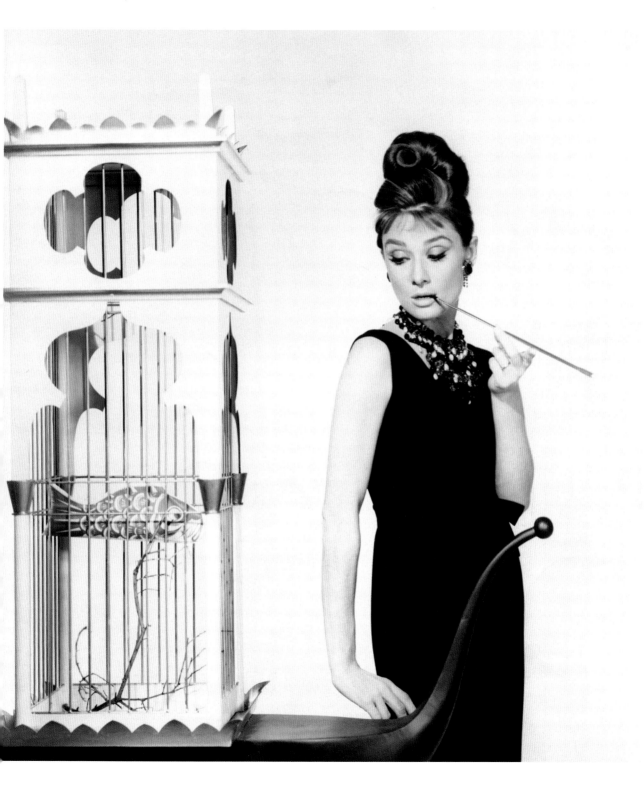

- **Bette Midler** played Mel Gibson's cannabis-imbibing psychotherapist in *What Women Want* (2000).

- Ganja is important to **Frances McDormand**'s free-spirited music producer character in *Laurel Canyon* (2002). McDormand tokes up on screen while trying to balance the stress of her career and coming to terms with her uptight son when he unexpectedly moves into her house with his fiancée.

- A disillusioned med student finds himself amid the marijuana farmers of California in *Humboldt County* (2008). This drama starring **Frances Conroy** and **Fairuza Balk**, who both regularly partake on screen, drags a bit, but has some nice moments and presents a somewhat realistic glimpse into a counterculture world most people never encounter.

- **Jane Fonda** is smoking again in *Peace, Love, and Misunderstanding* (2011), a generational comedy that also stars **Catherine Keener** as the uptight daughter of Fonda's marijuana-growing 1960s-era matriarch. It seems the two became estranged when Fonda's character sold weed at her daughter's wedding, and little has changed when mother is reunited with her daughter and granddaughters years later, after the daughter's divorce.

- **Blake Lively** is the pot-smoking protagonist who propels the action in Oliver Stone's marijuana-themed drama *Savages* (2012). Although it bears little resemblance to the reality of the American cannabis world, *Savages* does show a gruesome glimpse into the havoc prohibition has wreaked south of the border. For pure entertainment value, though, this tense drama about a pair of U.S. pot growers whose shared girlfriend is kidnapped by a Mexican cartel delivers . . . right up until the end—but I won't give that away.

Although the following are not stoner flicks per se, here are some favorite movies to watch while "under the influence." Gather some friends, make a batch of potcorn, heat up the vaporizer or fire up the bong, and enjoy some great home entertainment. Mary Jane can improve almost any favorite film—or any mediocre film, for that matter.

Oh, and don't forget to show a cartoon before the main feature! Any classic Looney Tunes segment will have everyone in stitches.

MARY JANE'S MOVIE-STAR FANS

- Activist **Susan Sarandon** has vocally spoken out against the drug war and the mass incarceration problem it has caused and is in favor of legalization. She serves on the advisory board of the Marijuana Policy Project and recently told *AARP* magazine, "I would much rather my kids smoke weed than drink, except that it's illegal."

- Always outspoken about her marijuana use, **Whoopi Goldberg** even publicly admitted to being high when she accepted her 1990 Oscar. Whoopi still loves her weed, penning a column for *The Cannabist* in 2014 entitled "My Vape Pen and I, a Love Story."

- **Frances McDormand** appeared on the April 2003 cover of *High Times* magazine holding a joint. In the interview she admitted to being a recreational pot smoker and went on to remark, "There has never been enough of a distinction between marijuana and other drugs. . . . It's a human rights issue, a censorship issue, and a choice issue."

- **Lily Tomlin** came out of the cannabis closet in the pages of *Culture* magazine, which asked the actress and comedienne if she supported marijuana legalization. Her answer? "Yes, of course."

- *The National Enquirer* published pictures of Oscar-winner **Charlize Theron** smoking from an apple pipe back in 2002.

- **Cameron Diaz** has never been shy about her marijuana use. She's been photographed smoking on several occasions, once passing a joint to *Charlie's Angels* costar **Drew Barrymore**, and opened up to *GQ* magazine about her pot-smoking surfer days while growing up in Southern California.

- While on a promotional tour for *Spiderman 3*, leading lady **Kirstin Dunst** told Britain's *Live* magazine, "I do like weed. If everyone smoked weed, the world would be a better place."

- TMZ caught **Kristin Stewart** toking away on her porch. The *Twilight* star was also photographed wearing a bikini that sported two strategically placed pot leaves on the top.

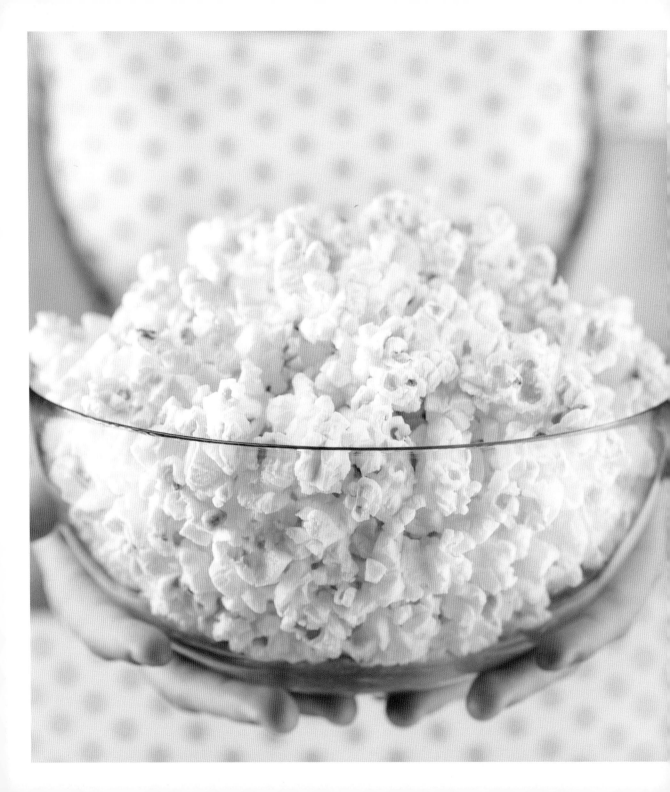

Second Childhood

You may not be a kid anymore, but kid movies are still fun to watch. These family-friendly films contain enough visual stimulation and/or oddness to make them even better (as Jon Stewart's character in *Half Baked* would say) "on weeeeeeed."

- *The Wizard of Oz* (1939). The world's best-loved children's classic can be even more fun when you're stoned; just make sure to get a nice mellow indica. Those flying monkeys can be really unnerving! Whether you opt for the original or the one with the Pink Floyd soundtrack (see sidebar "The Buzz: Great Stoner Bands"), you're guaranteed a great time.

- *Willy Wonka and the Chocolate Factory* (1971) or *Charlie and the Chocolate Factory* (2005). Your preferred version will likely depend on your age, but both the Gene Wilder original and the Tim Burton remake with Johnny Depp have enough color and high weirdness to keep adults highly entertained.

- *Alice in Wonderland* (2010). The whole story of Alice is already like a weird trip. Add the influences of Tim Burton and Johnny Depp, not to mention Helena Bonham Carter as the freakishly huge-headed Red Queen, and it gets even trippier. Add weed and get ready to be transported through the looking glass!

- *Chitty Chitty Bang Bang* (1968). The film version of Ian Fleming's book about a magical flying car has panoramic scenery, lively musical numbers, and enough bizarre characters that a little bit of ganja can take this kid's flick, which has always played second fiddle to *Mary Poppins* (also not bad to watch stoned), to interesting new heights.

Visual Extravaganzas

These movies all share breathtaking scenery or visually stunning sets and cutting-edge art design that with a little help from Mary Jane can transport viewers into an astounding other world for a few hours. In addition to the suggestions below, almost any film considered an "epic" could qualify for this category. Consider movies like *Gone with the Wind*, *Braveheart*, or *The Last Emperor*.

- *Moulin Rouge* (2001). Baz Luhrmann's over-the-top spectacle about a poor poet (Ewan McGregor) who falls in love with a French courtesan (Nicole Kidman) assaults the senses with stunning visuals of a highly stylized and romanticized

Paris of the late 1800s set to a rocking modern soundtrack.

- *Eyes Wide Shut* (1999). Stanley Kubrick's last film received a lot of attention when it came out for its scandalous sex scenes and the fact that it starred then husband and wife Tom Cruise and Nicole Kidman in the most no-holds-barred roles of their careers. One of his most visually lavish and erotically charged movies, it makes a good pairing with the tips from Chapter 10.

- *March of the Penguins* (2005). Smoke a nice bowl of indica, get mesmerized by nature's astounding dance, and prepare to be taken through emotional highs and lows in this riveting documentary, coproduced by the National Geographic Society, chronicling the annual single-file Antarctic march made by Emperor penguins to their traditional breeding ground. The soothing voice of Morgan Freeman tells the dramatic tale of life and death faced by these amazing birds, instinctually driven each year to face unimaginable hardships in the quest to ensure their species lives on.

Documenting the Truth

Documentaries represent some of the highest-quality movies made about marijuana. You'll find a wide array to choose from, covering an array of topics from prohibition, medical research, and drug war injustices and waste to political efforts to legalize, and more.

These films make it easy to learn the facts about this often misrepresented and misunderstood plant. They also make a great way to help friends and family learn the truth. Some pot-using parents have even used documentaries to introduce their kids to the subject of cannabis.

- *420* (2014). Filmmaker Amy Povah, herself a victim of the drug war who escaped nearly a decade of incarceration only after President Bill Clinton granted her clemency, does a commendable job of showing how the war on weed has corrupted and perverted our justice system. Povah's technique of juxtaposing the celebratory side of marijuana with the dramatic reality of lives ruined by drug raids and the mass incarceration of nonviolent marijuana offenders, some serving life sentences, illustrates the absurd reality of the times we are living through as prohibition falls, but not quickly enough.

- *American Drug War 2: Cannabis Destiny* (2013). As one of the latest documentaries about marijuana in America, the follow-up to filmmaker Kevin Booth's groundbreaking *American Drug War: The Last White Hope* focuses exclusively on cannabis and encompasses the game-changing legalization of recreational marijuana in Colorado and Washington state.

- *What If Cannabis Cured Cancer* (2010). This film explains, in a layperson's terms, how cannabis works in the body with a special focus on studies and research into its potential cancer curative abilities. It also goes into what the U.S. government knows and its cannabis patents, discusses cannabis-based pharmaceutical medicines, and provides a detailed look at the cannabinoids most intriguing to scientists and doctors.

- *a/k/a Tommy Chong* (2006). Real-life examples of how absurd, unjust, and wasteful the "war on drugs" has become don't get much better than what comedian Tommy Chong went through over some bongs (not marijuana, bongs) sold over the Internet. Not only was Chong set up and entrapped into the charges filed against him, but his subsequent prosecution and incarceration were clearly meant to make an example of him and to serve as retribution for his public decades-long pro-pot counterculture persona.

- *Waiting to Inhale: Marijuana, Medicine and the Law* (2005). An excellent documentary exploring both medical marijuana and the laws that effect it and the patients who depend upon it.

- *Grass* (1999). While this entertaining history of America's war on weed, narrated by Woody Harrelson, stops short of California's 1996 legalization of medical marijuana, it's one of the best and most engaging looks at this complex subject up to that point.

MARIJUANA IN YOUR LIVING ROOM—TOKING ON TELEVISION

Mary Jane's role on the small screen has definitely evolved since its reefer madness low during the 1980s and 1990s. Back then, the government actually paid television shows to put antidrug messaging into their plotlines. The results were embarrassing preachy propaganda pieces that now command the ridicule they so deserve.

For instance, then first lady Nancy Reagan made a "very special" appearance on the hit TV show *Diff'rent Strokes* in 1983 to help spread her "Just say no" message.

That episode spawned a host of other "very special" episodes on other family shows like *Full House*, *Family Ties*, and *Growing Pains*. Everyone's favorite cartoon characters even got in on the act of teaching America's kids all the "wonderful ways to say no" during a 1990 once-in-a-lifetime collaborative effort that accomplished the impossible and featured Disney characters romping around with Looney Tunes characters, Muppet Babies, and other revered animated figures, all in the name of keeping kids off "drugs." And in this era, the drug discussion always started with demonizing marijuana.

Nowadays, it's far more common to see marijuana use portrayed realistically as a normal part of events, as it is in the lives of millions of real cannabis consumers, whether for medicinal or recreational use. It may seem like cable shows are leading the charge, but the networks have been on board all along.

In 1997, Murphy Brown's then scandalous use of marijuana to treat her cancer outraged drug czar Thomas Constantine. Lots of other shows dealt with it in a neutral or positive light through the years, including *Roseanne*, *Home Improvement*, *Parenthood*, *Glee*, and *How I Met Your Mother*.

To be sure, the number of television shows that make marijuana the primary or even secondary focus are far fewer in number than movies that do so. Nonetheless, there are some good ones, and others in which marijuana is regularly part of the background.

- Weed is just part of everyday life for Fiona Gallagher (**Emmy Rossom**) and other characters in Showtime's *Shameless* (2011–).

- Mags Bennett (Emmy winner **Margo Martindale**) oversees a huge illegal weed empire in the FX series *Justified* (2010–). In a later season, lead character Raylan Given's girlfriend is a pot-smoking agent for Child Protective Services.

- Gemma Teller Morrow (**Katey Sagal**) regularly indulges for medicinal and recreational reasons in FX's *Sons of Anarchy* (2008–).

- Female leads Karen and Marcy (**Natascha McElhone** and **Pamela Adlon**) toke up in Showtime's *Californication* (2007–2014), as do a host of other characters, male and female.

- It has been fairly common for women to smoke marijuana throughout the course of AMC's *Mad Men* (2007–). In season 1, **Rosemarie DeWitt** plays lead character Don Draper's pot-smoking Greenwich Village beatnik girlfriend. In later seasons Draper (**Jon Hamm**) also smokes with his wife Megan (**Jessica Paré**),

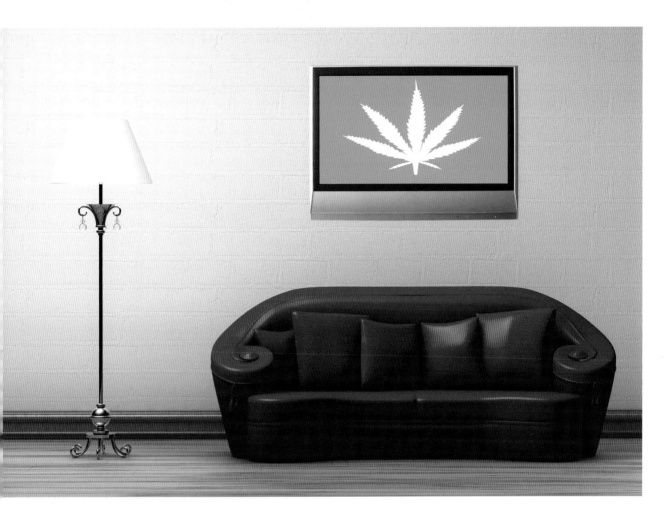

who scored the weed for them while on vacation in Hawaii. Copywriter Peggy Olson (**Elisabeth Moss**) also gets in on the action starting in season 3, when she proudly declares, "I want to smoke some marijuana."

- **Mary-Louise Parker** stars as Nancy Botwin, a suburban housewife who

turns to dealing marijuana to make ends meet after the death of her husband in Showtime's *Weeds* (2005–2012), although she never actually smokes cannabis until the very end of the series.

- On HBO's *Six Feet Under* (2001–2005), many of the leading and supporting characters smoke weed, including

Brenda (**Rachel Griffiths**), Claire (**Lauren Ambrose**), Ruth (**Frances Conroy**), and Bettina (**Kathy Bates**).

- While you don't actually see the characters use marijuana in Fox's *That '70s Show* (1998–2006), a sitcom about a group of 1970s-era Midwestern teenagers, the show usually begins and ends with the gang, including **Laura Prepon** and **Mila Kunis**, philosophizing in Eric Forman's smoke-filled basement. One episode also features Kunis's character scoring a bag of weed.

What the Doctor Ordered

TV cannabis is not all about getting high— America's acceptance of the medicinal use of marijuana is showing up more frequently on the small screen too. A 2013 episode of the CBS drama *Hawaii Five-0* starred octogenarian **Carol Burnett** as a medical marijuana-using cancer patient. On Showtime, **Edie Falco** in *Nurse Jackie* goes behind her hospital's back in order to score a sick patient some marijuana. And **Laura Linney**'s terminally ill cancer patient shares cannabis with her husband in Showtime's *The Big C*.

The medicinal side of marijuana is also on prominent display in the Discovery Channel's reality show *Weed Wars*, which chronicled life at the nation's largest medical marijuana dispensary, Harborside Health Center in Oakland, California. The short-lived series' most powerful episode revolved around the moving story of a young child racked by violent seizures who becomes nearly seizure-free with the help of medical marijuana.

Even the news has been jumping on the green bandwagon. All the major news networks have done specials on the growing legal marijuana industry. In addition, CNN's chief medical correspondent **Dr. Sanjay Gupta** made a very public apology to the world in 2013 for misleading them about marijuana. The former anti-cannabis neurosurgeon admitted he had been duped into believing the government propaganda. Gupta had his epiphany while researching a CNN special on medical marijuana. When he witnessed young Charlotte Figi being cured of debilitating convulsions by cannabis, he could no longer deny the truth and or stand silent about the government's interference in medical and scientific research. In 2014 Gupta doubled down on marijuana and came out with *Weed 2* to explore the subject further . . . or for ratings.

WEED IN YOUR EARS: MARIJUANA MUSIC

Since before prohibition, Mary Jane has been faithfully serving as a musical muse to generations of musicians. That's right, even in your grandparents' and great-grandparents' days, they were enjoying marijuana music! And new songs singing her praises come out all the time.

Instead of giving you the usual tired old list of "Top 10 Stoner Songs," I thought it might be fun to create some different playlists. Well, not completely different. All of them—regardless of genre, style, or subject nuance—pay homage to everyone's favorite herb.

Oldies Are Goodies: Boogie Down with the Grandparents (and Great-Grandparents)

Tons of marijuana songs graced the airwaves in the 1930s, and 1940s, and even earlier. A lot of them were instrumentals with titles that gave a wink and a nod to those "in the know," while the lyrics to others left nothing to the imagination. Your grandparents might have danced the night away to some of these songs on their dates. Here are some of my favorite tokin' tunes of yesteryear.

- "Reefer Man" (1933). A fun and funny fast dance number dedicated to the crazy antics of a favorite stoner by **Cab Calloway and His Cotton Club Orchestra** and featured in the film from the same year, *International House*.

OUT OF THE CANNABIS CLOSET: *TV Stars*

- **Roseanne Barr** likes marijuana so much she ran for president of the United States on a legalization platform.

- **Sarah Silverman** has been and continues to be outspoken about her marijuana use, talking about it in her act and even smoking onscreen with Doug Benson in the film *Super High Me* (2007).

- Not only did comedienne **Joan Rivers** spark one up on her reality series *Joan and Melissa: Joan Knows Best?* (2011–2014), but when TMZ asked her who else she had smoked with, she spilled the bong water and outed **Betty White, George Carlin, Woody Allen**, and **Bill Cosby**.

- Back when she was still married to **Brad Pitt**, **Jennifer Aniston** told *Rolling Stone* that she smoked marijuana and saw nothing wrong with it, and, in fact, she and Pitt frequently smoked together.

- **Martha Stewart** admitted in an interview with Andy Cohen that of course she knew how to roll a joint. During a 2013 *Today Show* appearance, Martha quipped that she and Snoop Dogg hang out together and bake brownies. Stewart has even spoken out publicly about the need for sentencing reform, especially for nonviolent drug offenders.

- Sweet little **Mary Ann (Dawn Wells)** of *Gilligan's Island* fame was busted with marijuana in the car in 2008.

HOW TO:

Fun with 420

A friend and I came up with a game in which we take a puff every time marijuana gets mainstream media coverage. Toke up every time you hear it mentioned, chuckle at a subtle pot reference, or see an onscreen character light up. In an evening of normal television watching, you'll be smoking more than you might think.

Another fun game is "spot the 420." Yes, some of America's television writers must be fans of ganja (gasp!). If you pay attention, you can find frequent 420 references in a lot of shows, and movies too, for that matter. Look for the number and you'll catch it popping up on hotel room or apartment doors, street addresses, flight or train numbers, meeting times, and a host of other innocent and coincidental spots.

- "That Cat Is High" (1938). The **Ink Spots** provide great harmonies in this classic that has been covered by countless artists through the decades. Check out the **Manhattan Transfer** version for a modern take that leaves the song's retro tones solidly intact.

- "Do You Dig My Jive?" (1941). **Sammy Price and His Texas Bluesicians** create a sultry, jazzy ode to the history and pleasures of "jive," a.k.a. cannabis.

- "The Spinach Song (I didn't Like It the First Time)" (1947). A fun, danceable tune about the lead singer's growing fondness for "spinach" by **Julia Lee and Her Boy Friends**.

- "Marijuana Boogie" (1949). Old-time jazz got a Latin flavor with **Lalo Guerrero**'s south-of-the-border classic.

- "Sweet Marijuana" (1976). Originally recorded in 1934, **Bette Midler**'s cover is even better than the original and far easier to find.

Free the Weed!

The ending of prohibition has been a long battle that has yet to be completely won. A lot of artists have weighed in on the subject with protest songs in musical styles as diverse as the people who use cannabis.

- "Safe in My Garden" (1968). Gorgeous harmonies underscore this amazing **Mamas and Papas** track that contrasts the safety of the garden where "an ancient flower blooms" with the turbulent protests, police actions, and times of the late 1960s. Best of all, it's just as relevant today.

- "Don't Step on the Grass, Sam" (1968). Another 1960s song that is just as relevant today is this Steppenwolf tune that

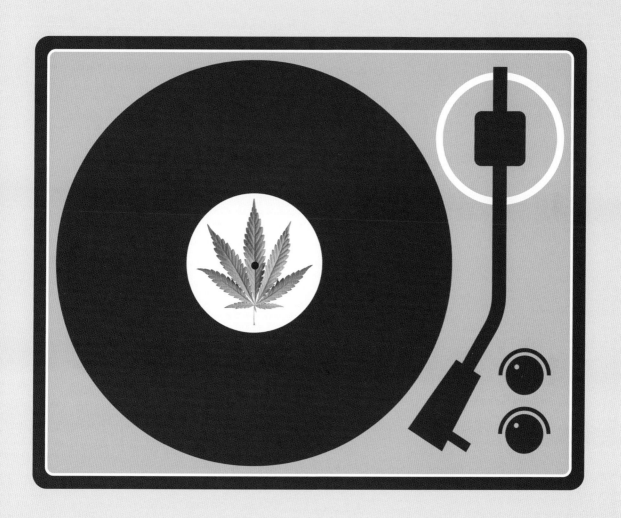

> ## HOW TO:
> ### *Build Your Marijuana Music Library Fast!*
>
> Do a search on any popular music source under the word "marijuana" and you'll be rewarded with a variety of collections dedicated to the herb in various genres, including vintage music, reggae, rock and roll, and hip-hop. These make for a quicker and less expensive way to build a large marijuana music collection, rather than buying individual songs.

talks back to mainstream TV's prohibitionist talking heads.

- "John Sinclair" (1971). **John Lennon** wrote and performed this song at the John Sinclair Freedom Rally (and on his *Some Time in New York* album) in December 1971 to protest the sentencing of poet and political activist John Sinclair to ten years in prison for the "crime" of giving two joints to some undercover narcotics officers. Three days after the rally, the Michigan Supreme Court ruled the state's marijuana statutes unconstitutional. Sinclair was released. The event inspired the Ann Arbor Hash Bash (see Chapter 14) that continues to this day.

- "Legalize It" (1976). **Peter Tosh**'s reggae classic, his first solo effort after leaving

The Wailers, has become an anthem for the marijuana movement.

- "(Hey, Uncle Sam) Leave Us Pot Smokers Alone" (1982). Playful and lighthearted yet brutally honest in its politics, this **Toyes** song will get the whole crowd to enthusiastically sing along at your next party.

- "Burn One Down" (1995). "If you don't like my fire, then don't come around, cause I'm gonna burn one down," **Ben Harper** sings in this unapologetic declaration on the virtues of ganja.

- "Legalise Me" (1999). "I'm just a farmer and I grow marijuana," sings **Chrissie Hynde and The Pretenders** in this rocking anthem to freedom.

- "Can Anybody Hear Me?" (2008). The **Kottonmouth Kings** use hip-hop to express the frustration every marijuana advocate encounters when dealing with prohibitionists in this powerful track.

- "A Fire Burns for Freedom" (2010). **Ziggy Marley** sees "hemp fields forever" and "marijuana trees growing wild and free" in this utopic vision of a perfect world when we "unchain these wings and let angels fly!"

- "Play the Greed" (2012). Singer-songwriter **Dar Williams** creates a beautiful folk protest song for the new millennium with nods to legalizing hemp and marijuana, among other crucial American issues like solar power, destruction of natural resources, and corporate control of the media.

What the Hell Just Happened?

You know how your friends like to talk about that time that they had the really super-great weed and they got soooooo stoned? Yeah, well, so do musicians.

- "One Toke over the Line" (1970). In this country-tinged hit, **Brewer & Shipley** sang about sitting in a railway station while being "one toke over the line." For a good laugh, Google the unintentionally kitsch version, performed by **Dick Dale** and **Gail Farrell** in 1971 on the *Lawrence Welk Show*.

- "Panama Red" (1973). All manner of mayhem is likely to happen when "Panama Red is back in town," warned the **New Riders of the Purple Sage** in this classic stoner favorite.

- "Two Hits and the Joint Turned Brown" (1976). The weed was so good that **Dillard, Hartford, and Dillard** added a

bit of gospel style to their bluegrass in this fun song that invariably inspires a sing-along when you hit the chorus.

- "Weed with Willie" (2003). **Toby Keith** musically expounds on the experience most of us can only dream of: smoking marijuana with the great Willie Nelson.

- "Blueberry Yum Yum" (2004). A love song to the "ultimate Mary Jane that will put your stuff to shame." Exercise caution when smoking Blueberry Yum Yum because, as **Ludacris** warns, it might cause you to eat everything in sight!

Say It Isn't So!

Not only can good marijuana inspire good music, but so can the lack of it. These songs all sing the woes of what every marijuana user knows as a "dry period."

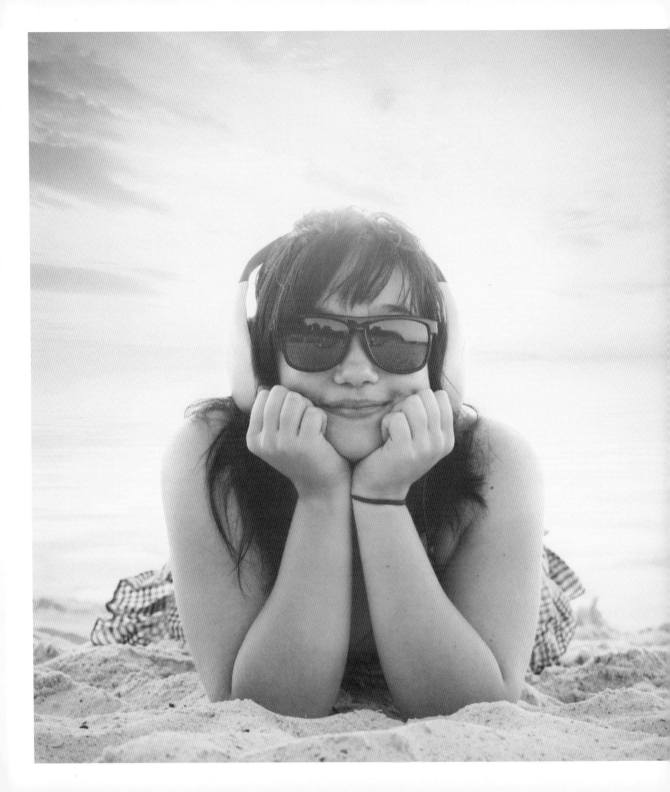

- "Little Green Bag" (1970). Even though the **George Baker Selection** is frantically searching for that lost "Little Green Bag" in this 1970s hit, judging from this song's upbeat tempo, they sure seem happy about it.

- "Henry" (1971). A dry period inspired the **New Riders of the Purple Sage**'s "Henry" to head to Mexico for 20 kilos of Acapulco Gold. The rest is musical legend.

- "Down to Seeds and Stems Again Blues" (1974). Things don't get much worse than being down to seeds and stems, but at least you'll have **Commander Cody and His Lost Planet Airmen** to commiserate with.

The Joy of Marijuana

For those times when you are looking for a happy escape, the feel-good songs in this list celebrate the pure joy of cannabis. Sometimes that exuberance takes the form of carefree youthfulness, sometimes it's spiritual, and sometimes it's just plain fun.

- "Rainy Day Women # 12 and 35" (1966). As my best friend's elderly grandfather observed in a thick Russian accent while driving down the road with **Bob Dylan**'s oompah band rhythms blaring out the windows, "That's a catchy little tune." Everyone sings (even Grandpa), "I would not feel so all alone; everybody must get stoned!"

- "Stoned Soul Picnic" (1968). While the cover versions by the **Jackson 5** and **The Fifth Dimension** might be better known, composer **Laura Nyro**'s original celebration of a summer picnic enhanced by Mary Jane is still the best. Surry on down!

- "I Like Marijuana" (1968). You won't find any slick production in this comedic **David Peel & the Lower East Side** track, but, if you play it, expect everyone in the room to start singing about how much they like marijuana too! My favorite line: "Make me president and I promise you a pot in every chicken!"

- "Marijuana" (1969). **Country Joe and the Fish** sang about how much they liked marijuana and how much they sure did like to get stoned way back at Woodstock. I bet they still do.

- "Sweet Leaf" (1971). Metal heads will find no finer love song to Mary Jane than the hard-pounding rhythms of **Black Sabbath**'s smoking hot "Sweet Leaf."

- "Wildwood Weed" (1974). This is a playful little tune about some country boys

THE "LOUIE LOUIE" OF WEED SONGS

It's speculated that "Louie Louie" is the most covered song in the world. Rhino Records even released two entire volumes of nothing but "Louie Louie" covers. The weed world's answer is "Smoke Two Joints." So many folks have played this song, there's now a version for everyone, no matter your musical genre preference.

The song originated in 1982 with **The Toyes**. According to the band's website, the first night they performed "Smoke Two Joints," they had to play it five more times because the crowd kept interrupting other numbers by chanting "Smoke Two Joints" louder than The Toyes could play.

Knowing a good thing when they heard it, the band not only recorded the song in English but covered themselves by also recording in Spanish (*Dos Leños*) and French (*Fume Deux Joints*).

To be sure, you can find more versions than those listed below. My favorite is still The Toyes' reggae original, but here are some other interesting musical takes on smoking two joints:

- **Sublime** (1992). The most famous version, many people mistakenly believe the ska-punk infused Sublime take on the song to be the original.

- **Richard Cheese** (2002). "America's Loudest Lounge Singer" offers up arguably the most creative "Smoke Two Joints" cover, with a beautifully orchestrated big-band Vegas-style interpretation of the song that first makes you laugh before making you say, "Hey this is really good!"

- **Norman Nardini** (2009). Pittsburgh's "unknown King of Rock and Roll" gives the "two joint" experience a bluesy rock spin featuring a smoking-hot guitar solo.

- **Filthy Freqs** (2012). The song is barely discernable in this deep bass techno, dubstep version, but, if techno is your thing, check it out.

- **Macy Gray** (2012). Although it's a pretty direct cover of the Sublime cover, Macy Gray's husky vocals give her version a certain smoky authenticity.

- **Fish Fry Bingo** (2013). Billed as "pure raw hillbilly," Texas band Fish Fry Bingo give the song an outlaw country spin with washboards and rocking banjos (yes, banjos CAN rock!).

harmlessly enjoying the freely growing weeds on the farm until the feds ruin the party . . . sort of. A mainstream crossover hit for **Jim Stafford**, "Wildwood Weed" charted at number 7.

- "Granny Wontcha Smoke Some Marijuana?" (1976). Bring this smokin' fiddle-laden **John Hartford** bluegrass ditty out at your next barn dance and get ready for the fun to start!

- "Planet of Weed" (2007). **Fountains of Wayne** fantasize about what life could be like on their utopian vision of an entire planet of marijuana in this light-hearted pop song.

- "Live High" (2008). **Jason Mraz** gets introspective and spiritual in this glorious tribute to living "high and mighty, living righteously, and taking it easy." Abide on, Jason.

- "San Disco Reggaefornia" (2010). **Jason Mraz** likes weed. Here he will be passing out the "high-fives" (you know, the medical kind) in "San Disco Reggaefornia," a joyful ode to the best of California culture.

- "Dieman Noba Smoke Tafee" (1997). The perfect world music accompaniment to a mellow afternoon buzz, the title of this meditative track by Sierra Leone's **S. E. Rogie** translates to "Dead Men Don't Smoke Marijuana," although there are no lyrics to the late guitar virtuoso's almost instrumental track that would give that away, at least not in English.

- "Roll Me Up" (2012). **Willie Nelson** gets some help from Snoop Dogg, Kris Kristofferson, and Jamey Johnson in the ultimate funeral song that begs Willie's mourners to simply roll him up and smoke him when he dies.

Pass It Already!

"Puff, puff, pass" is the proper sequence of events in a stoner circle. Nonetheless, some people just don't get it and need to be reminded. Try one of these musical hints to keep the doobie moving!

- "Don't Bogart Me" (1968). Also known as "Don't Bogart That Joint," this was the biggest hit for **Fraternity of Man** when a place on the *Easy Rider* soundtrack put the song into the nation's consciousness.

- "Light Up or Leave Me Alone" (1971). This rocking **Traffic** song expresses a possible remedy to a frustrating stalled relationship.

- "Pass the Kouchie" (1981). The Jamaican trio **The Mighty Diamonds** originally sang about passing the kouchie, or pipe, from the left-hand side in this reggae classic.

- "Pass the Dutchie" (1982). British group **Musical Youth** incorporated big parts of "Pass the Kouchie" in their 1982 reggae hit "Pass the Dutchie," further cementing the practice of passing to the left-hand side.

- "One Draw" (1990). "Hey Rasta Man, give me some of your sensi," **Rita Marley** joyously sings. Why? Because she wants to get high, of course!

- "Pass It, Pass It" (2004). "You're supposed to take two puffs, then give the shit up," raps **Snoop Dogg** in this track backed by **Pharrell Williams** and **Vanessa Marquez**.

Weed Will Get You Through

Sure, marijuana makes the good times even better. But it can also get you through the rough periods too, as these musical tributes attest. A lot of them are surprisingly upbeat, considering the emotions and situations they deal with, but cannabis does have a way of making it easier to cope with negativity.

- "Reefer Blues" (1970). Mope around or feeling down all day? **Canned Heat** has some advice that can help you chase your blues away.

- "Willin'" (1971). The road can be a lonely place when you're making long hauls, but "weed, whites, and wine," always made **Little Feat** "Willin'" to keep on moving. Be sure to check out Linda Ronstadt's cover on her *Heart Like a Wheel* album.

- "Roll Another Number (for the Road)" (1975). In this song written after the death of two friends from drug excesses, **Neil Young** is consoled by "rolling another number for the road," making him feel he could "get under any load."

- "Kaya" (1978). Even though the rain was falling, **Bob Marley** knew that "Kaya" would make him feel good and "so high I can even touch the sky."

- "Family Tradition" (1979). "If I get stoned and sing all night long, it's a family tradition," is **Hank Williams Jr.**'s explanation for his wild ways in this classic country anthem.

- "Champagne and Reefer" (1981). There are a some great earlier versions of this classic blues song, especially by **Muddy Waters** and **Mojo Buford**, but for my money the best version is by the **Rolling Stones** backed by, as Mick Jagger calls him, **Buddy "Motherfucker" Guy**.

- "Electric Avenue" (1982). Despite poverty and violence in the streets, **Eddy Grant** knows you can always "Rock on Down to Electric Avenue" to get higher in this reggae crossover hit.

- "What I Got" (1996). No matter how bad things got, **Sublime** sang about retaining the ability to "still get high." Whew! It will all be OK as long as "lovin' is what you've got."

- "To Be Young (Is to Be Sad, Is to Be High)" (2000). A lot of folks will relate to **Ryan Adams**'s twangy, bluesy ode to youthful dramas and their most popular remedy.

- "Because I Got High" (2000). OK, maybe **Afroman** is actually blaming marijuana for his lack of progress in this lighthearted hit, but, judging from the tone of the song, he's not too upset about it. "La da da da da, shoop-shoop shoobey do wah!"

- "Hash Pipe" (2001). A hash pipe provides the only solace for a male prostitute working his trade on Santa Monica Boulevard in this hard-hitting **Weezer** track.

- "Smoke a Little Smoke" (2009). **Eric Church** brings a sultry spin to country pop with this bluesy tune that sings the praises of turning the quiet up and the noise down with the help of a couple of favorite substances.

- "Marijuana" (2010). That "pretty green bud" is "the only thing that keeps me level up in my crazy head," claimed **Kid Cudi** in his love song to cannabis. After all, it's always had his back and never left him lonely.

- "Hush Hush" (2013). **Ashley Monroe, Miranda Lambert,** and **Angaleena Presley,** collectively known as **Pistol Annies,** sing about relieving pressure at a tense family Christmas gathering by sneaking out for a toke behind the barn.

- "Follow Your Arrow" (2013). **Kacey Musgraves** encourages listeners to follow their arrows wherever they point, including "rolling up a joint, or don't" (Kacey would) when the "straight and narrow gets a little too straight" in this boppy country feel-good song from her Grammy-winning album *Same Trailer Different Park.*

- "Dark Sunglasses" (2014). There's a whole lot of smoking going on in the video for **Chrissie Hynde**'s song that references how Mary Jane can help people get through their workaday lives.

Mary Jane in Love (or Lust)

Love inspires a huge percentage of songs, so it stands to reason that some great marijuana songs would be dedicated to the subject as well. Here's the playlist for Chapter 10.

- "Mary Jane" (1978). Who knew that "Super Freak" **Rick James** was actually a one-woman man? He is unabashedly in love with Mary Jane (and he's "not the only one"), whether she can love him

WOMEN ROCKING OUT OF THE CANNABIS CLOSET

They may or may not sing about marijuana, but these music stars are definitely out of the cannabis closet.

- **Miley Cyrus** is a fan of marijuana leaf fashion in her personal AND professional lives. She wore a bejeweled costume covered with marijuana leaves on tour and famously blazed on stage during the European Music Awards. The singer has been and continues to be outspoken about and unapologetic for her marijuana use.

- **Melissa Etheridge** openly supports and has campaigned for legalization, and has even appeared in a documentary about her experience using marijuana therapeutically during her battle with cancer.

- In a *60 Minutes* interview, **Lady Gaga** admitted, "I smoke a lot of pot when I write music." She has even been known to smoke a giant prop joint on stage. Then she came out saying she was "addicted to pot" but has since backpedaled, telling British talk show host Alan Carr how much she loves smoking marijuana because it makes her feel seventeen and forget that she's famous.

- Always outspoken about social causes, **Chrissie Hynde**, lead singer of The Pretenders and rock goddess in her own right, has come out in favor of legalization, appeared on the cover of *High Times* magazine, and even penned the song "Dark Sunglasses" (see "Weed Will Get You Through" playlist).

- **Alanis Morissette** confided to *High Times* magazine, "As an artist, there's a sweet jump-starting quality to [marijuana] for me. So if ever I need some clarity . . . or a quantum leap in terms of writing something, it's a quick way for me to get to it."

- Music icon and fashionista **Rihanna** has been frequently photographed smoking herb and wearing pot-leaf-embellished clothing. Both Ri-Ri and Lady Gaga have celebrated Halloween in marijuana-themed costumes.

- Rock icon **Patti Smith's** book *Just Kids* describes how she sees pot more as an aid to her work than a social drug.

- Songstress **Joss Stone** has taken a lot of heat in the British tabloid press for her candor about her own marijuana use. Depending on what she is working on, Stone says, she sometimes uses the herb every day. She has also preached the marijuana-is-safer-than-alcohol mantra.

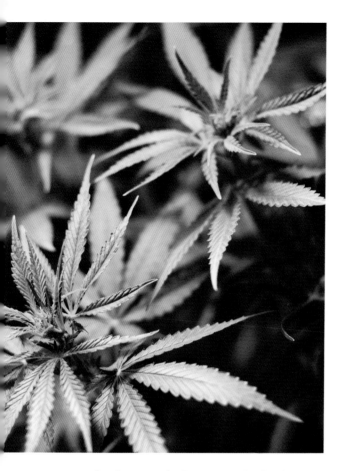

> " I'd take out a joint and light it. First just faking it, then I started lighting live joints, passing them around to the band, you know. It was great, it relieved all my tensions. "
>
> —*Barbara Streisand to Rolling Stone*

- "Take a Toke" (1994). **C&C Music Factory**, the same folks who brought you the frenetic "Everybody Dance Now," lets you slow down and get close with this sexy tribute to marijuana's sensuous pleasures.

- "High" (2004). **James Blunt** celebrates the glory of life, love, and being high in this joyous song. "Promise me that tomorrow starts with *you* getting high!"

- "Weed Instead of Roses" (2013). **Ashley Monroe** defines romance for the modern country couple by spicing up the relationship with whiskey instead of wine, and weed instead of roses, 'cause heaven knows we don't need another box of chocolates!

back or not. (Side note: Rick's backup singers on his 1979 tour were known as the "Mary Jane Girls.")

- "Reefer Head Woman" (1979). **Aerosmith**, fronted by Steven Tyler's sexy screaming vocals, pays homage to a "Reefer Headed Woman who fell right down from the sky" (Good Lord!) in this hard-rocking blues number.

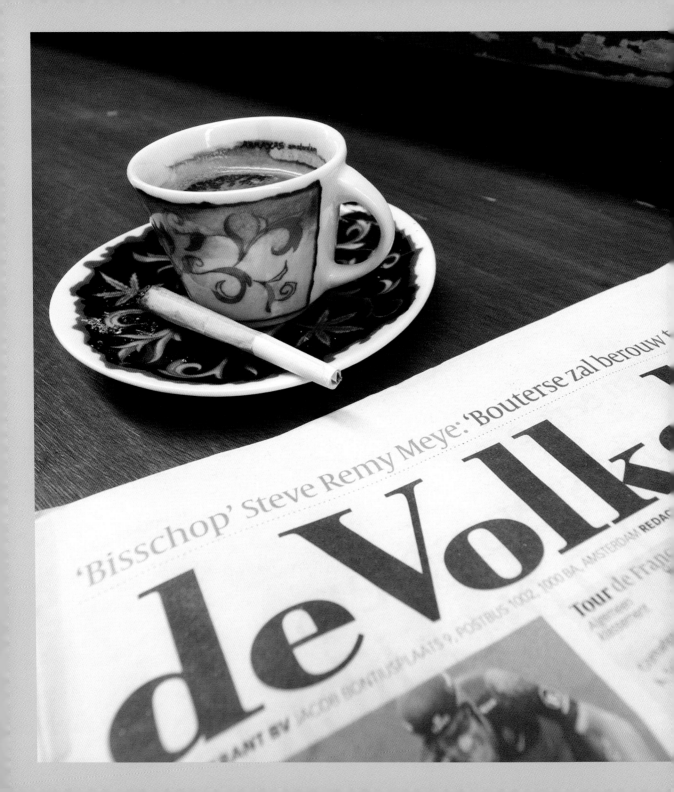

CHAPTER 14

HOP *on the* CANNABUS: TRAVELING *with* MARY JANE

To some degree, cannabis tourism has been around for a long time. After all, for decades tourists have been flocking to Amsterdam to easily and openly procure marijuana. Thanks to the loosening of marijuana laws, there are now more opportunities than ever to incorporate marijuana into your leisure time travels and activities right here in the United States.

Before we get into all the great places and fun events you can visit, let's look at the practical side of traveling with marijuana in your possession because nothing can ruin a vacation more than arrest and jail time.

FLYING HIGH: THE PRACTICALITIES OF TAKING WEED ALONG

Your medical license to consume marijuana in your own state will not impress nonlegal states or the federal government. Exercise caution when transporting or possessing cannabis where you are not legally allowed to do so.

The same goes for flying, especially internationally. As you will recall from Chapter 5, airports are one of the few places where officers are allowed to search you and your possessions without a warrant.

For the record, the Transportation Security Administration states that its procedures focus on security and are designed to detect potential threats to aviation and passengers. If TSA agents discover illegal items in the course of a search, they will turn them over to law enforcement.

Regardless of the official stance, I know of countless instances when the TSA agents let both patients and medicine pass without incident. This is especially true for travel within legal states and between legal states. But since their official policy states otherwise,

MEDICAL MARIJUANA RECIPROCITY

Does your medical marijuana state have *reciprocity* with others? I checked with Dale Gieringer, an attorney and director of the California branch of the National Organization for the Reform of Marijuana Laws (NORML) for the current policies. Like anything marijuana-related, there is no one easy answer, and policies can change from year to year, so always check for updated information.

- Arizona, Montana, and Rhode Island offer medical marijuana reciprocity with other medical marijuana states.

- Maine will allow out-of-state visitors to exercise their medical marijuana rights for thirty days.

- Michigan will accept out-of-state cards but ONLY from other states that have reciprocity, so if yours doesn't, you are out of luck in the Wolverine State.

- Vermont will accept medical marijuana recommendations from neighboring states but ONLY if you are a Vermont resident.

- Oregon does not offer reciprocity, but it does allow out-of-state patients to register with the Oregon Medical Marijuana Program to obtain a registry identification card, which will protect against arrest or prosecution while in Oregon.

Always keep in mind that, even though you are in a state that offers reciprocity, within its borders you must observe that state's medical marijuana laws. These laws might differ substantially from those of your own home state. Check out the details before traveling.

it is always up to the individual officer on a case-by-case basis, so you never know.

If you plan on driving with marijuana, be sure to review Chapter 5 for tips on how to avoid legal problems and what to do if you are stopped by law enforcement.

THE WORLD OF CANNABIS: AMSTERDAM AND BEYOND!

When you talk about marijuana and world travel, all thoughts immediately go to Amsterdam. Yes, cannabis is technically illegal in Holland, but it never seems to be enforced. Even recent rumors that the Dutch government was cracking down on sales to foreign tourists have not resulted in any change in the coffee shop cannabis trade.

So is it really as easy as going into a coffee shop and ordering marijuana right off the menu? Yes indeed it is. Nonetheless, here are some things first-timers should know about imbibing and ordering in Amsterdam:

- A lot of Europeans like to mix tobacco with their cannabis, so be aware that, if someone passes you a joint, there might be more in it than you are expecting.

- Amsterdam coffee shops are known for their fine selections of hash as much as they are cannabis flowers, so don't neglect sampling some while you are in town.

- This is Europe, which means you will be purchasing in grams, not ounces (or fractions of ounces).

The interiors of Dutch coffee shops and American medical marijuana dispensaries look different. They certainly give off different vibes—the dispensary often being clinical and minimalistic, the coffee shop warm, inviting, and social. Nonetheless, they share a few things.

- Dutch coffee shop staff, like good U.S. budtenders, know their merchandise and can be your best friend when deciding what to buy. Don't be afraid to ask questions and get their recommendations.

HOW TO:
Mary Jane Math Conversions

Do your math skills need a tune-up? Refer to this handy chart when ordering in Amsterdam (or most non-U.S. locales). While the *actual* conversions are a fraction of a gram higher than what's listed, in practice the amount is always rounded down to the closest ½ gram, so that's what's given:

- 1 ounce = 28 grams
- ¼ ounce = 7 grams
- ⅛ ounce = 3.5 grams

Both the coffee shop server and budtender should know about indicas, sativas, and their effects, along with the quality and characteristics of what is currently in stock.

- As in U.S. dispensaries, it is OK to look at and even ask to smell the cannabis before buying in the coffee shop, but it is NOT OK to touch it.

- As a general rule, pre-rolled joints in both scenarios will be made from shake or lesser-quality cannabis.

HOLI FESTIVAL

A springtime Hindu festival celebrated in the north of India, *Holi* is known around the globe as a celebration of colors because everyone plays with water guns and colored powders. The best part? Government-sanctioned vendors selling marijuana-laced drinks and sweets. Yes, cannabis is illegal in India, but drinks like Bhang Lassi (see Chapter 10) are so ingrained in the culture and religion that officials take the pragmatic approach of "if you can't beat 'em, join 'em."

According to April Price, an international travel expert and cannabis tour coordinator based in New York City, there are lots of other places around the world where anyone can easily score marijuana, whether it's legal or not. Once I got April talking, she had both great destinations to share and tips on how to delicately broach the subject.

April Price's Tips for International Cannabis Travelers

- Best countries to score weed (other than Holland): Canada, Jamaica.

- Best cities/regions to score weed (other than Amsterdam): Barcelona, Prague, and the surf towns of Australia, such as Nimbin.

- Honorable mention domestic location: the "hippie" beach town of Pa'ia on the island of Maui, where you should also seek out Little Beach on Sundays for some awesome drum circle action starting at 4:20 PM.

- The best people to approach for scoring weed: bartenders in hip areas, student tour guides, people sporting dreadlocks.

- The best places to score weed: vintage vinyl record stores, open-air markets, beach resorts, anywhere near a surf or snowboard scene.

- Wearing a small pot leaf somewhere on your apparel helps a lot, according to April, giving people silent confirmation that you're "cool."

EXPOS AND FESTIVALS

A weekend at a marijuana festival will immerse you in cannabis culture. While each festival has a slightly different focus and personality, all of them share some common features:

- **Vendors.** You'll get a far better deal on things like pipes, vaporizers, and all manner of cannabis accouterments and accessories at an expo than you ever will at a typical retail outlet. Depending on the event, you may also

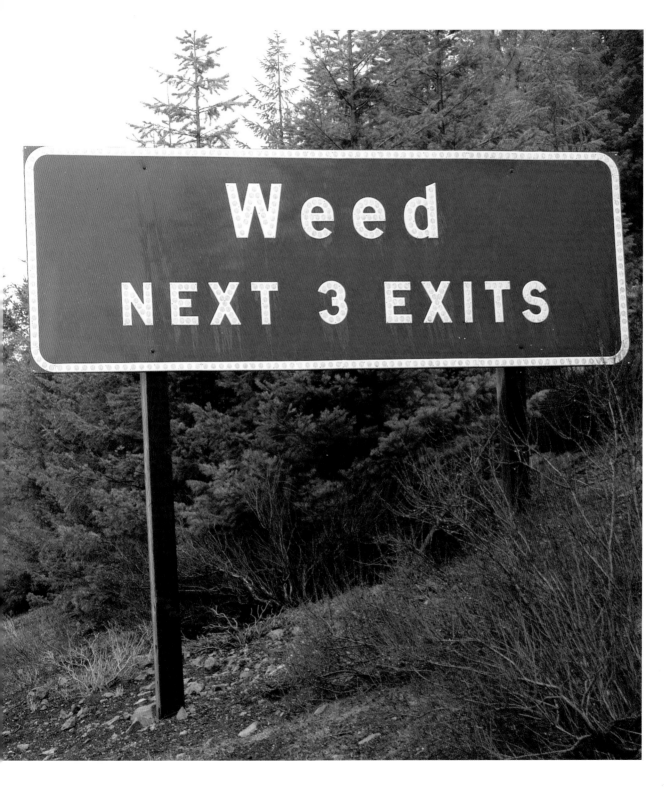

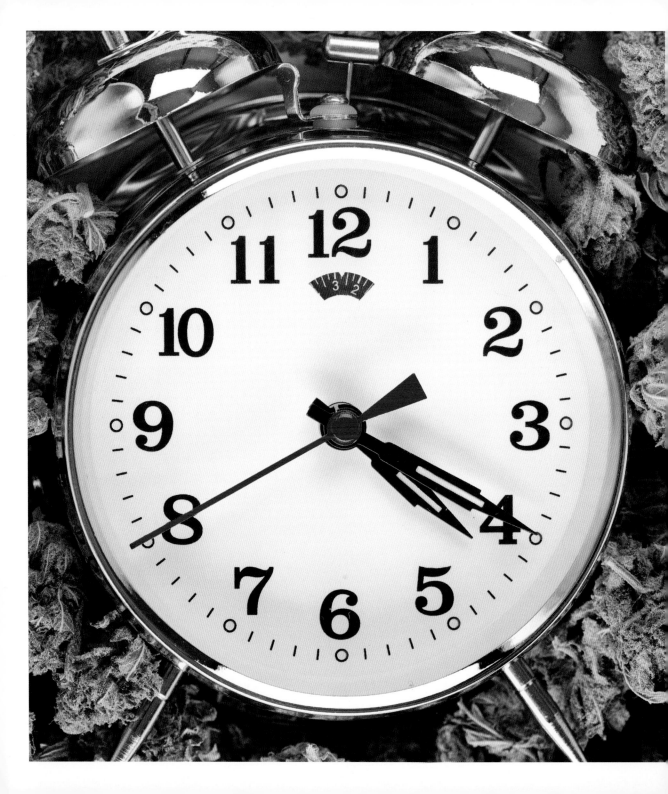

see demonstrations of all the latest products, from small smoking accessories to options for a large-scale grow operation.

- **Lectures and panels.** Further your cannabis education by attending lectures and panel discussions on a variety of topics like growing, edibles, policies and politics, health, and more.

- **Doctor's recommendations.** Many shows in medically legal states will have doctors on-site to write medical marijuana recommendations.

- **Competitions.** Some festivals include a competitive component in which growers, concentrate makers, and edibles manufacturers compete for prizes. While you, the consumer, won't get to actually sample all the entries, you will learn where to find the best marijuana and marijuana products, and sometimes the entry products are available for purchase.

- **Medication area(s).** In legal and medicinally legal states, shows will also set up an area where you freely ingest marijuana in public and with your friends. Bring your doctor's recommendation and ID along in order to access these areas and, depending on the event, to be able to purchase marijuana, concentrates, edibles, and plants.

> " It's always 4:20 somewhere, right? "
>
> —*Sarah Silverman*

- **Entertainment.** Many of the bigger and better expos feature one or more big-name musical acts.

Depending on where you live, you may be inundated with so many expos you'll burn out on them. Los Angeles, Denver, San Francisco, and Seattle all have more than their fair share throughout the year. Other areas are starving for these kinds of events. If you need to travel to experience a cannabis expo, here are some good ones to consider. Some of them are even free to attend!

- **High Times Cannabis Cups.** You get at least five chances per year to attend a High Times Cannabis Cup. Even though this famous event began as an annual competition in Amsterdam, it has now evolved into a series of competitions and festivals held annually in Los Angeles, San Francisco, Seattle, and Denver, as well as the original Amsterdam. *High Times* events are always well attended and always feature some excellent educational panels along with all the fun. www.cannabiscup.com

- **Seattle Hempfest.** Held each year on the third weekend in August, the size and scope of this volunteer-run Seattle event has grown with the expanding legal marijuana movement into the mother of all marijuana events. Since it is held in a public park, there is no admission fee and typically hundreds of thousands of cannabis enthusiasts attend the festivities, which always include compelling speakers and kick-ass musical guests. www.hempfest.org

- **Portland Hempstalk.** Founded in 2005 by the Hemp and Cannabis Foundation, the festival takes place in September. Attended by some 30,000 people, Hempstalk can be thought of as a smaller, more intimate, and friendlier version of Seattle's Hempfest. Free admission. www.hempstalk.org

- **The Emerald Cup.** Started as a small mid-December harvest festival in California's "Emerald Triangle" of Humboldt, Mendocino, and Trinity counties, this event moved south to Sonoma in 2013 to the larger venue of the county fairgrounds. Event producers accomplished the impossible and kept the grower-centric harvest fest vibe while expanding the show to include more panels, vendors, and some first-rate

musical guests. Unique among competitions, only outdoor organically grown cannabis and concentrates extracted without solvents qualify for entry. You'll find that the Emerald Cup is one of the best shows for true connoisseurs and serious marijuana enthusiasts. www.theemeraldcup.com

- **Ann Arbor Hash Bash/Monroe Street Fair.** The country's oldest annual marijuana rally, the Hash Bash began after the Michigan Supreme Court ruled that the law used to convict legendary activist John Sinclair (see Chapter 13) of giving two joints to undercover officers was unconstitutional. You can always expect some inspiring speakers during the Hash Bash, which is held on the University of Michigan campus, and some great music and partying at the adjacent Monroe Street Fair. Best of all, these events are free. www.monroestreetfair.com

- **Boston Freedom Rally.** The East Coast's answer to Seattle Hempfest, albeit with somewhat less free-flowing weed, the Freedom Rally has been fighting with the city of Boston for its right to exist (and winning) almost since its inception in 1989. The event has moved a number of times, growing and thriving in the process, and is now an annual,

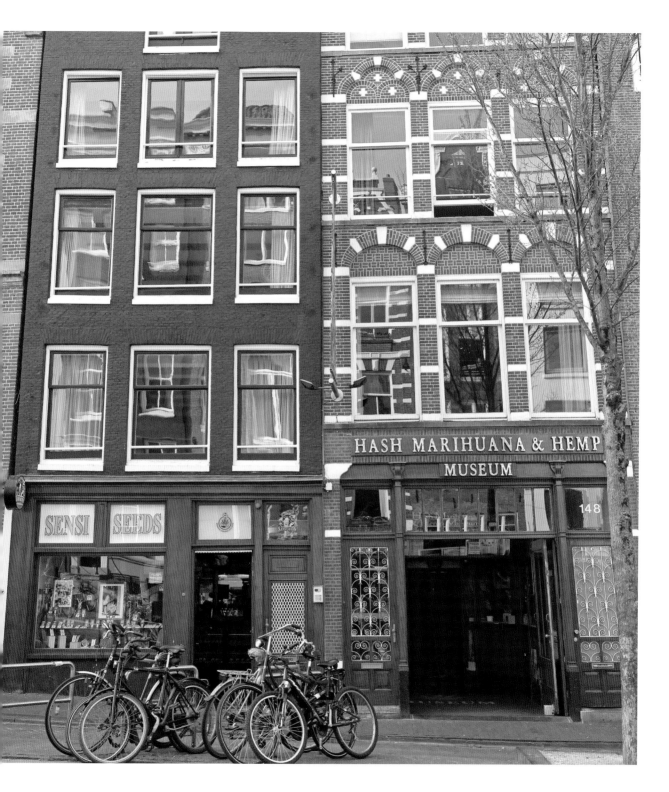

HAPPY 420!

As more and more states loosen marijuana laws, April 20—aka 420, the "Stoner's Holiday"—is growing by leaps and bounds each year, including coverage by major news outlets. April 20 has become a day to celebrate all things ganja.

The origins of the number are a constant source of debate in the cannabis community, with each raconteur claiming he or she knows the actual, bonafide truth about how it all began. The most popular version has a group of Marin County, California, high school students meeting each day after school for the daily toke party at, you guessed it, 4:20 PM.

High Times regularly holds its Denver Cannabis Cup during 420 week, but, even without the cup, the Mile High City always hosts a robust outdoor 420 party right in front of the state capitol building. When the witching hour hits, a thick sweet-smelling smoke cloud hangs over the entire area.

You'll also find parties, festivals, and events taking place all over the country on April 20. A good place to check for places to celebrate is your local alternative weekly newspaper, or with your local NORML chapter.

April 20 only comes around once a year, but there are plenty of opportunities to celebrate year-round: marijuana enthusiasts the world over regularly spark up at 4:20 PM each day.

free, two-day festival held in September. Visitors can expect compelling speakers, great music, lots of vendors, and fun! www.masscann.org/rally

THE BUDDING U.S. CANNABIS TOURISM INDUSTRY

When I started writing this book, most cannabis tourism opportunities were underground. In other words, you had to know someone who knew someone to even find out about them. But things are already beginning to change, especially in states like Colorado and Washington, where adult recreational marijuana use has already been legalized. More hotels and inns are advertising the fact that they don't mind if their guests use cannabis.

Colorado seems to be blazing the trail. Visitors will find marijuana-friendly visitors guides and tour companies that offer 420-friendly food, lodgings, and activities. These tours make Colorado's already spectacular tourist offerings even better by adding marijuana to the mix, including visits to commercial grow operations, retail dispensaries, and cannabis cooking classes.

Cannabis-friendly lodgings and activities in medical marijuana states like Michigan, California, Oregon, and Washington (which also legalized marijuana for recreational purposes) are also starting to come out of the shadows.

Marijuana social clubs have begun to pop up in major cities. To be sure, the World Famous Cannabis Café in Portland, Oregon, led the way. Opened in 2009 by medical marijuana activist Madeline Martinez, this 4,000-square-foot facility where patients can gather, procure, and ingest marijuana offers everything a friendly neighborhood bar would, if you substituted marijuana for alcohol. Yes, you must show your medical card to get in, but Oregon has a program in which medical marijuana visitors from other states can register with the Oregon Medical Marijuana Program to obtain a registry identification card that will gain you access. Check their website for a schedule of events. www.usaworldfamouscannabiscafe.com

Things in the world of domestic cannabis travel are changing and evolving so quickly, a computer and a good search engine are the best planning tools to stay up-to-date.

Another good resource for travel to recreationally legal states can be found at www.cannavacation.com.

HIGH ON REFORM

Consider an education vacation. Attending a drug policy reform conference is a great way to get educated, meet and network with other

HOW TO:

420 Travel Game

Here's a fun little travel game. See how many times you can spot the number 420 during your travels. Once you start looking, you will see it everywhere. On hotel room doors, street addresses, plane and train schedules, price tags, and more. I always like to snap a photo for my 420 album!

individuals who share your values, and have fun at the same time. NORML puts on an annual conference at varying locales that features great speakers, workshops, and parties.

Every other year, the Drug Policy Alliance (DPA) brings reform leaders and activists from all over the world together for a conference jam-packed with outstanding seminars, brainstorming sessions, and workshops addressing all aspects of drug policy reform. Check with these organizations for upcoming conferences you might like to attend.

Even regionally and locally you will find reform events, often put on by chapters of national organizations, that can bring you up to speed with what is happening in your immediate area and how you can help.

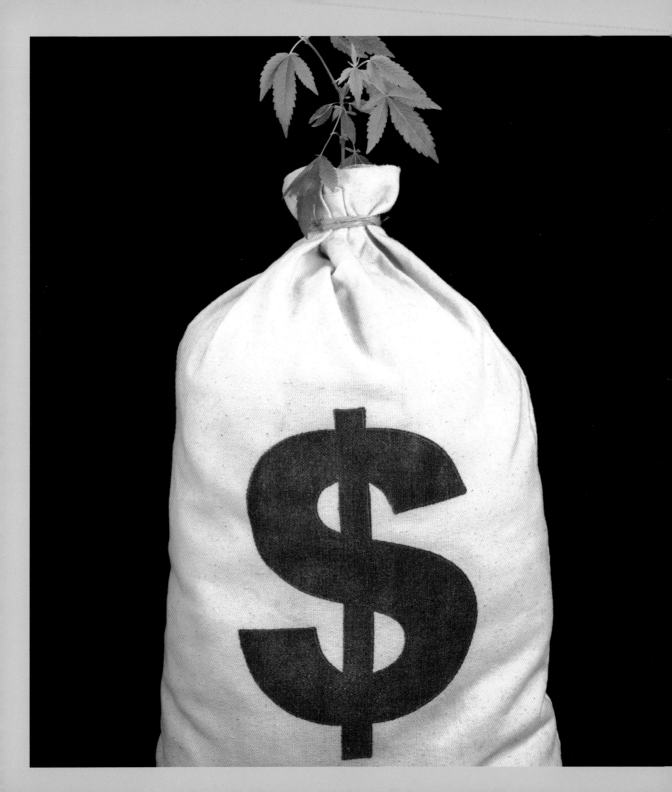

CHAPTER 15

KUSHY JOBS: CAREERS *in the* CANNABIS INDUSTRY

Making money with Mary Jane is not just happening on *Weeds* anymore. All those parents who told their kids they would never amount to anything smoking weed all day might just have to eat those words! The fact is, marijuana is America's number one cash crop and plenty of people make plenty of money in the weed business, and, yes, a lot of them actually do smoke weed all day. And a lot of them don't. If you want to work directly in the legal cannabis industry, consider these careers (but not before you thoroughly read Chapter 5).

- **Dispensary/collective/cooperative operators and/or caregivers.**
  Depending on where you live, you may call yourself any of these names (and probably a few more) for legal reasons. But the bottom line is this position involves overseeing a system

for distributing marijuana to qualified patients (or, in states where recreational marijuana is legal, qualified adults). That entails managing the actual facility and its employees or volunteers, sales, accounting, taxes, legal matters, security, and procurement of inventory. The latter may or may not involve managing a grow operation. Some states require collectives to grow their own, others strictly prohibit this practice, and still others leave it up to the individual.

- **Delivery service operators.** Even though you won't maintain an actual brick-and-mortar shop, your cannabis delivery service will still likely be called by the names in the first point above. This job will also entail all the duties above, with the exception of maintaining the facility, but has the added responsibility of physically delivering the marijuana to the customer's/patient's door.

- **Budtenders.** The service personnel who work behind the counter at marijuana dispensaries, good budtenders should have a good working knowledge of cannabis. Because budtenders are the people who interact most with the public, it also helps if they are familiar with the collective's available strains and their properties so they can help people make the right choices for their needs.

- **Growers.** Somebody actually has to grow all that marijuana! Collectives, dispensaries, and delivery services depend on growers. Sometimes collectives grow their own, but more often than not they procure their cannabis from growers. The size of these grow operations can range from small home gardens all the way up to warehouse-size industrial grows. If you grow high-quality weed, someone will want to buy it. Be aware that most collectives will not bother with any amount under a half pound and will generally require more. Some growers may specialize in seeds, clones, and/or breeding new strains.

- **Buyers.** Large-scale dispensaries require a lot of cannabis to meet the needs of their patients, and they may employ a buyer to help fill those needs. The buyer must have an extensive knowledge of cannabis along with a connoisseur's palate, much as a wine sommelier does with wine. The buyer's job includes procuring the best-quality cannabis at the best prices. This includes the ability to identify strains along with flaws like mold, age, poor curing, pests, and more.

- **Grower's services.** Most growers take care of these tasks in house, but as the industry grows we are seeing more and more discreet services aimed at making the grower's job easier and more profitable, such as trimming and making hash and oil. Of course, you will see a greater proliferation of such services in areas that produce a lot of marijuana, such as California's "Emerald Triangle" (see Chapter 14) and Colorado. If you know people who grow, you know they almost always need help around harvest time, especially if they grow one large outdoor crop. Get in with the right people and you can always find freelance trimming work in areas that grow a lot of outdoor cannabis. Some enterprising individuals have set up trimming services that provide an entire professional, bonded crew that gets the trimming job done quickly, neatly, and discreetly. Turning those trimmings into hash or oil (see Chapter 3) is another great grower service business an entrepreneurial individual with the right connections could offer.

- **Marijuana products manufacturer.** As we discussed earlier, there are lots of ways to ingest cannabis. Likewise, there are lots of jobs to be had producing products such as edibles, concentrates, and topicals, of which the variety is endless.

ANCILLARY MARIJUANA CAREERS

An old business rule says that, in a gold rush, you should sell shovels. The same applies to the cannabis "green rush." Besides the obvious careers working directly with marijuana, ancillary careers that support the industry allow you to be involved without the same level of risk. Here are just a few of the industries, businesses, and jobs that stand to increase our country's employment numbers as the cannabis industry grows and more people jump on the legalization bandwagon:

- **Medical.** We have barely scratched the surface of medical marijuana's potential, yet already the industry employs

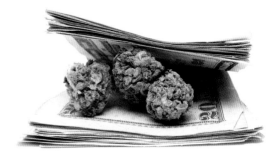

doctors, nurses, technicians, clinic managers, and the support staff it takes to maintain medical offices.

- **Science.** Marijuana-testing labs are already big business and as prohibition ends and the government's monopoly on research loosens, more grants and funding are likely to become available, meaning more demand for scientifically accurate testing and research in the public, private, and academic sectors.

- **Legal.** As complicated as the nation's drug laws have become, the need for criminal attorneys isn't going away anytime soon. The industry also supports a host of civil and business lawyers along with their support staffs, including secretaries, paralegals, investigators, and expert witnesses.

- **Financial.** As the cannabis industry transitions from underground to "legitimate," the need for banking and merchant services will grow, especially because the federal government has intimidated many banks into not working with the industry. This is beginning to change, but, wherever there is a need, there is opportunity.

- **Building/construction.** Every marijuana dispensary and grow needs some build-out, including people who specialize in carpentry, plumbing, and electrical.

- **Security.** Dispensaries need security systems and on-site security guards and may need armored cars to move the money.

- **Property rental.** Whether it's a small storefront dispensary, a commercial kitchen to manufacture edibles, or a huge industrial grow operation, cannabis businesses are always in need of 420-friendly landlords.

- **420-friendly care facilities and living options.** Seniors represent the fastest-growing demographic in the cannabis market, which only makes sense as cannabis is one of the best weapons against aging. As legalization expands, people will be looking for cannabis-friendly places to live, both for medical care and in general. Cannabis-savvy landlords and assisted care facilities stand to cash in.

- **Media, marketing, and public relations people.** Marijuana is big news and it takes a lot of publishers, writers, radio, video, and Internet people to get the word out. Opportunities abound in this niche, from working with the mainstream media to becoming an independent blogger and everything in between.

- **Artists/photographers.** The above media empire will need logos and other art along with great photography to help tell the story. All the budding entrepreneurs entering the wonderful world of cannabis business will also need these services, along with packaging design for their products.

- **Printers.** Marijuana enterprises will need business cards, stationery, packaging, and more. All those cannabis publications that are sprouting up like mushrooms in legal states will also need someone to print, produce, and distribute them.

- **Technology services.** Like other businesses, marijuana industries need website design and consulting, search engine optimization, mailing list management solutions, and telephone communications services.

- **Professional services.** Business insurance, property insurance, health insurance, retirement and investment plans, and more—people in the cannabis business will need these products.

- **Trade organizations.** This is a brand-new industry that can benefit from like-minded people working together for their mutual benefit.

- **Suppliers.** Nutrients, hydroponic equipment, lighting, growing medium, grow tents, pots, fans . . . the list of garden supplies goes on forever, and somebody has to supply all those things to the gardeners and to the stores that sell to the gardeners.

- **Inventors, craftspeople, and entrepreneurs.** Visit any cannabis show, whether consumers or trade, and you'll be greeted by an astounding array of clever (and sometimes not-so-clever) marijuana-related gadgets and products . . . but there's always room for more.

- **Event producers.** The legal and quasi-legal states already host a dizzying array of marijuana shows and expos, but there's always room for a creative producer to succeed with another. Plus, new territory opens up all the time. You could even host educational expos in states that have not yet legalized marijuana.

- **Educators.** Who is going to supply the employment needs of this industry? Those who educate others. Classes, schools, and seminars, whether online or in person, present opportunities for the right people, whether you teach at an already established institution, or market your own knowledge.

- **Travel and recreation.** Still in its infancy, the legal marijuana travel industry is expected to be huge. Tour operators, 420-friendly travel services, hotels, restaurants, clubs, and more all offer potential income streams.

MARIJUANA U: TRAINING FOR CANNABIS CAREERS

In the early days of the legal cannabis movement, if you wanted to learn about marijuana, you went to Oaksterdam University. The first cannabis college in the country was founded in 2007 by Richard Lee, who played a big hand in revitalizing a formerly derelict part of downtown Oakland with cannabis businesses.

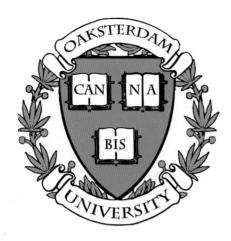

Now run by Dale Sky Jones, Oaksterdam is still a hub of activism and a great place to learn all about marijuana and marijuana businesses. Students have the choice of enrolling to study a full curriculum exploring all the options, or concentrate on areas that interest them, such as comprehensive grow seminars. OU also offers a certification program if you're applying for a job in the industry. Their curriculum offers what you want to know to thrive and, more importantly, what you didn't realize you needed to know.

Medical Cannabis Caregiver's Institute in Pasadena, California, is another good place to learn. It not only features first-rate guest instructors but is actually approved by the California Department of Social Services to teach the state Medical Marijuana Program under the CDSS ongoing Education Program for Licensees and Administrators

of State-Licensed Residential Care Facilities. It's the only school in the country with such credentials. Another MCC benefit is that, once students have paid to take a course, they are welcome to come back and repeat it as often as they like, giving them ongoing access to experts who can answer questions and concerns at later dates.

As the industry has grown, other schools, seminars, and classes have emerged. Some are rooted in a single location; others are mobile. Some even offer online training. Some are excellent and led by true masters in their fields. But like any highly misunderstood subject, the cannabis world has attracted more than its share of hucksters and con artists who are out to make a quick buck. Beware because a lot of these folks can be found selling seminars.

So how can you tell the good from the bad? Do a little research first and pay attention to these points.

- How long have these educators or institutions been in the industry? What are their credentials? What have they accomplished?

- Beware of anyone who says, "If you do it my way, there will be no risk of prosecution." No matter how confident a teacher is, this is simply not true. I have heard many a slick salesperson make this pitch. Educating yourself can lessen your

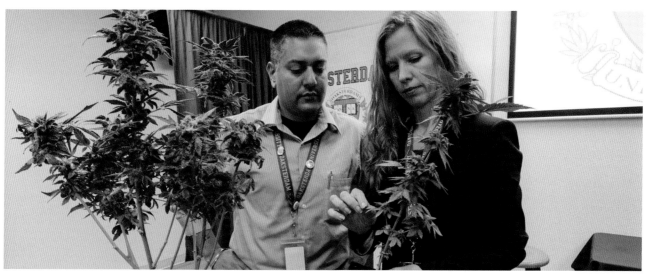

▲ *Oaksterdam University chancellor Dale Sky Jones (right) examines a marijuana plant at the school's Oakland campus*

chances of legal troubles, but as of this writing, you cannot eliminate the risks.

• Do an Internet search for the instructors and/or the company. Be sure to keep looking to page 3 or 4 of your search. For example, I know of a couple of extremely high-profile cannabis "entrepreneurs" who get lots of media coverage. At first glance, the public seems to adore them. But if you do a tiny bit of digging, you'll find a cornucopia of nefarious activity and little in the way of actual accomplishments. Dig a little deeper than usual before laying out any money.

• What is the instructor's or company's reputation within the industry? Again, do a little digging. Facebook is a good place to look. Don't necessarily believe the person's own press. Do a Google search too and see what kind of stories or posts come up. Again, be sure to glance through to page 3 or 4 at a minimum.

• If you are researching a school, check out online reviews of the school, talk to references, and make inquiries of consultants.

• Look up teachers' credentials and reputations.

• Do the same for administrative staff.

• Is the school or the educator/consultant involved with any cannabis reform efforts and/or organizations? They should be.

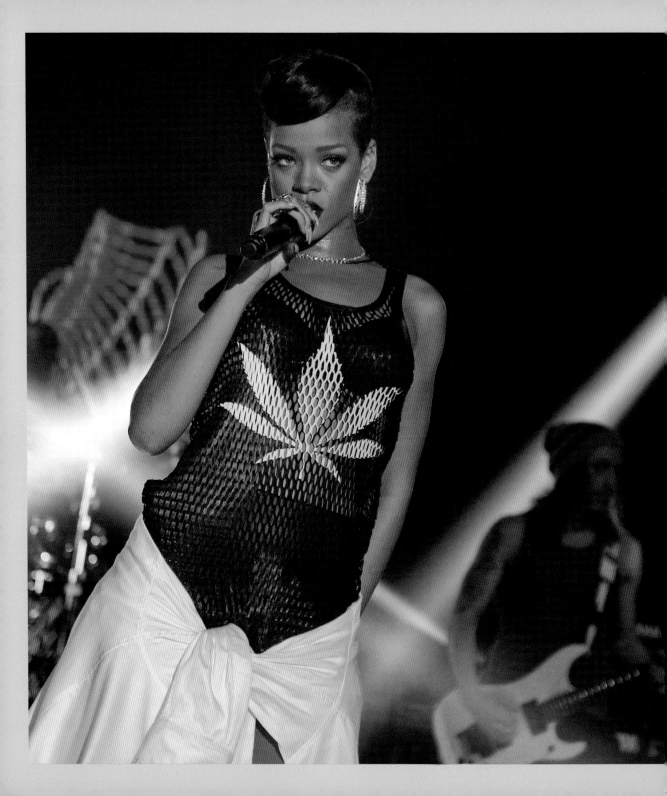

CHAPTER 16

YES WE CANNABIS!
BE *an* OPEN ADVOCATE

While some of you have every reason for not being open about your cannabis use—for instance, you fear losing your job, student loans, or public assistance, or you're afraid that this information will give a vindictive spouse something to use against you in a custody battle—the more people are honest about their use, the quicker things will change.

There's a lot on the line. Think of these major positive implications if we ended prohibition once and for all. Legalizing marijuana would

- remove medical research roadblocks;

- offer a safe, natural, alternative therapy for hundreds of afflictions from minor to terminal;

- remove fear of arrest and prosecution for simple marijuana use or cultivation;

- remove fear of losing your children because of cannabis use, whether prescribed by a doctor or not;

- remove fear of losing jobs, public assistance, student funding, and so on;

- remove a major source of funding for drug cartels and organized crime;

- cripple the corrupt prison industrial complex;

- free resources and time for law enforcement to focus on serious crime;

- clear the court system of nonviolent marijuana "criminal" trials;

- stop incentivizing corrupt civil asset forfeiture proceedings against people who have NOT been charged with or convicted of any crime;

> " I'm posting pictures of myself smoking pot to tell the truth about myself. "
>
> —— *Rhianna*

- reduce alcohol use and traffic fatalities (see Chapter 17); and

- allow cultivation of renewable industrial hemp, which can be used to make over 20,000 products in a cleaner and less environmentally damaging way than we currently do, including plastics, paper, fabrics, architectural building materials, and, best of all, fuel!

To truly embrace the cannabis lifestyle, I encourage you to consider venturing outside the safety of your "cannabis closet" and speak openly about your use. Talking to others about cannabis—whether they are in your close circle of acquaintances, your local and political representatives, or the world at large—is one of the easiest forms of "activism" anyone can do to help end prohibition. For decades, the stigma associated with marijuana, not to mention fear of prosecution, has kept many people who in fact do support reform from ever voicing an opinion on the subject.

But old taboos and outdated opinions based on lies are giving way to the age of enlightenment. Well over half of all Americans support the legalization of recreational marijuana; for medical marijuana, that stat is well over 80 percent!

Most of us who have come out, myself included, report far less negative blowback than we ever anticipated. This issue crosses all boundaries—age, sex, race, religion, and political affiliations—so you are likely to find support in some unexpected places.

The reverse is also true. The friends and acquaintances who are against might also surprise you. For instance, I had a friend in the music and restaurant businesses that I was sure would be enlightened on the subject. To the contrary, he bought into the bogus "Marijuana is a gateway drug" theory hook, line, and sinker because he personally knew a heroin addict who used to smoke cannabis. No amount of scientific research was going to convince him otherwise. Period. End of story.

TALKING TO YOUR PARENTS OR GRANDPARENTS, OR EVEN COMPLETE STRANGERS, ABOUT MARIJUANA

Sometimes you just have to come clean. In my outspoken life, the last people I told were my much older, conservative, religious sister and brother-in-law. To my surprise, they were fine with it. That said, approaching someone you think, or even know, will disapprove of your marijuana use can be daunting. Here are some tips to keep in mind when taking the plunge.

- Be aware of generation gaps. Everyone living in the United States has been subjected to government-sponsored brainwashing, some of us longer than others. Some in advanced age groups may have a problem grasping the concept that everything they've been told is wrong. Cut them a little slack but never stop educating. Seniors are some of the best advocates and some of the people who can most be helped by the medicinal properties of cannabis.

- Be aware of cultural differences. Culturally and racially speaking, the fact remains that some groups lag behind others when it comes to polling on the legalization issue, including women, blacks, and Hispanics. Ironically, the latter two groups stand to lose the most by continuing prohibition because they are arrested and incarcerated in far greater numbers than their Caucasian counterparts (see sidebar). The reason behind this lag can often be attributed to the stigma of not wanting the group to be painted in a negative light because of marijuana use. Again, be sensitive to the issue but keep on educating.

- Be prepared. Know your facts, figures, and science. If you can make people understand the truth about marijuana, very few lack the intelligence to not see the light unless they have financial motivation to do otherwise (see Chapter 17).

- Be ready for follow-up questions and conversations. Depending on whom you talk to, you may have to have the conversation again. And again. As you can tell by the scope of this book, prohibition has turned a simple plant into a complex subject. It may take a while for some people to come around.

- Lead by example. If you want your family and friends to know how beneficial your cannabis use is, make sure you are presenting a good face. Personally, I love to tell people I am a "stoner," because it shocks them and makes them look at the word and the substance in a new way. But then people see me as a together, successful, independent woman. If you appear to be a burned-out loser who always flakes out on her responsibilities, you can't expect people to approve.

- If someone is determined to remain hostile, move on. Some people already have their minds made up and nothing is going to change them. NOTHING. This is one of the most frustrating situations a budding cannabis advocate will encounter, but there's nothing you can do about it. NOTHING. Give it your all and then move on to someone more receptive.

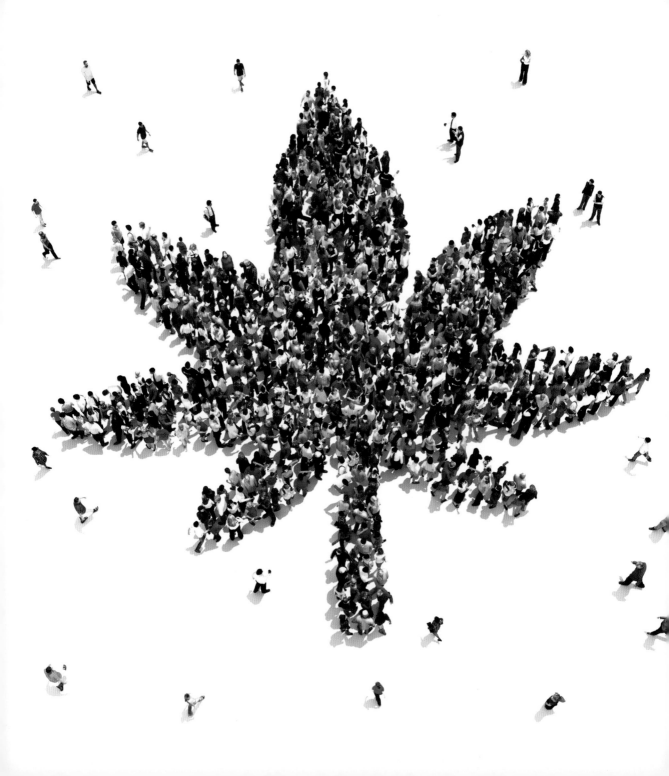

EASY WAYS TO HELP THE CAUSE FROM HOME

Even if you are not ready to jump in and become a full-on activist, there are lots of simple things you can do to help the cannabis reform movement from the comfort of your own home.

- Up the ante. If you're already out of the cannabis closet and being open about your support for the cause—and for a lot of folks this is an ever-evolving process—take it up a notch and start posting on social media. Sharing your experiences and credible news stories will help to educate others. We are near a crucial tipping point, and every person who comes to understand the truth puts us that much closer to ending the madness.

- Sign petitions. There are lots of online petitions dealing with cannabis (find them through the organizations listed in this chapter). Start signing them and sharing them. Depending on where you live, you may also get to sign petitions to put legalization measures on the ballot, although you will have to do those in person.

- Write to your elected representatives. The Internet makes it quick and easy to communicate with the people who represent you at all levels of government.

SHOCKING!

Reefer and Racism, the Modern Edition

Are marijuana arrests and prosecutions really racist? You decide. Based on federal data, *The New York Times* reported that black Americans were nearly four times as likely as whites to be arrested on charges of marijuana possession in 2010, even though the two groups used the drug at similar rates.

According to Ezekiel Edwards, director of the ACLU Criminal Law Reform Project, "State and local governments have aggressively enforced marijuana laws selectively against black people and communities, needlessly ensnaring hundreds of thousands of people in the criminal justice system at tremendous human and financial cost."

Make sure they know your feelings about cannabis. After all, your taxes pay their salaries, and, if enough of their voting constituents want something, politicians will take note.

- Write to the media. Once you learn the truth about cannabis, all the inaccuracies you'll see and hear in mainstream media stories will drive you crazy. Don't let them go unchallenged! Whether you send a letter to the editor or leave comments on an online story, let your voice be heard.

- Write to cannabis POWs. A lot of people are in prison because of the war on

Write to Marijuana POWs

Nobody should go to jail for a plant. That's the motto of The Human Solution (THS), an organization whose principal mission is to support those going through marijuana court cases and Child Protective Services abductions, as well as prisoners around the country paying the ultimate price for getting caught in the crosshairs of the war on weed.

THS volunteers maintain a list of people in prison for marijuana "crimes." The public can visit the Human Solution website, read the stories, and find addresses to write to the prisoners themselves. The Human Solution even has an "Adopt a Prisoner" program in which volunteers provide financial support and advocate for their adoptees.

For more information, visit www.the-human-solution.org.

weed. A card or letter from someone on the outside who cares and is paying attention can be one of the most powerful and meaningful pieces of mail you'll ever send (see sidebar above).

WORTHWHILE CANNABIS ORGANIZATIONS

A lot of dedicated, passionate people are working on cannabis reform, but not nearly enough. Personally I support most of the organizations below because I operate from the plain and simple belief that nobody should EVER go to jail for a plant, and the more people work on this issue from the more angles, the sooner it will get solved. You, however, may find that one or more of the following organizations fits better with your vision for the future of cannabis.

There is a group for just about everyone on this list, and it is by no means complete. In addition to the big national organizations, there are many small local chapters and organizations working to make change happen. You can usually find those in the calendar sections of many of the websites listed.

If, for some reason, there isn't a reform group within your area, you could always start one. National and international organizations can help you set up a local chapter wherever you live.

NORML, or the National Organization for the Reform of Marijuana Laws, is working for the day when recreational and medicinal use of marijuana will no longer be a crime. In addition to the national organization, there are numerous local chapters that approach the issue at the state and local levels.

The NORML Women's Alliance was formed to address the shortage of women in the movement and the fact the women typically poll between 5 to 10 points behind men on the issue of legalization. What began as an offshoot of NORML has now morphed into its own organization. NORML Women believe that prohibition is destructive to families and that the laws against marijuana cause far more harm than the substance itself and send mixed and false messages to our youth.

The members of Law Enforcement Against Prohibition (LEAP) include former and current police officers, judges, prosecutors, and other criminal justice professionals. These people have been on the front lines of the drug war and they know firsthand the harms it causes. LEAP speakers are visible warriors in the fight against prohibition, educating the public, the media, and policy makers. They know that the drug war has undermined the public's faith in law enforcement and work hard to promote policies that will help restore that faith.

Students for Sensible Drug Policy (SSDP) is an international network of college and university students who feel that the war on drugs is failing America's students and youth. The group encourages students to get involved in the political process and change the laws and policies that affect their lives and futures.

The Marijuana Policy Project (MPP), and its political arm the MPP Foundation, work to increase public support for legalization and lobby the policy makers who can help make it happen.

Based on the core belief that individuals should have sovereignty over their own minds and bodies, the Drug Policy Alliance (DPA) works on sensible policy for ALL drugs, not

GOTTA HAVE IT!
Safer Shirts

MARIJUANA IS SAFER THAN ALCOHOL. This simple message, boldly emblazoned across T-shirts, has been starting conversations throughout the country. Funds permitting, activist Jared Allaway will send you a T-shirt or a stencil so you can make your own T-shirts and signs. Allaway is doing this for free. Of course, sending Jared a donation for the shirt or stencil allows him to send out more shirts and stencils and keeps the message spreading.

Every time I wear my "safer" shirt, I am amazed at how well the message resonates with the public. Random strangers will come up and tell me they agree with what the shirt says, and more than once people have wanted to take their picture with me just because of the shirt. Get your "Marijuana Is Safer Than Alcohol" shirt at www.safershirts.org.

just marijuana. Its goal is to advance policies that reduce the harms of both drug use and of prohibition itself. In addition to its own programs, DPA grants also help fund other activism organizations and projects.

ACTIVISM IN THE JURY BOX

So many of us try hard to get out of jury duty, but, the fact is, you will never be in a greater position to effect change in the war on weed than by serving on a jury in a marijuana trial.

Most people serving on juries do not realize they have to the right to vote "not guilty" on

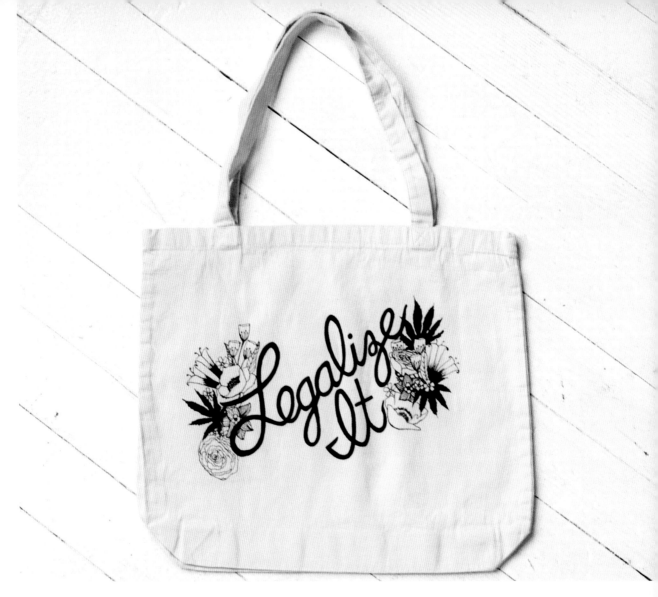

immoral laws. Judges and prosecutors are not likely to tell you this, either. In fact, they usually tell juries the exact opposite: "Even if you don't agree with the law, you must find the defendant guilty if you believe he committed the crime."

The concept of jury nullification started during the Civil War to protect those who refused to return runaway slaves to their owners, but it can also be used to protect marijuana users and providers. The simple fact is

SHOCKING!

Life Sentences for Nonviolent Marijuana Crimes

You might think the headline above refers to some Third World country, but the fact is there are many people in the United States, right now, in prison for life without possibility of parole for nonviolent marijuana "crimes." These people are the victims of conspiracy laws, mandatory minimum sentencing, and the courts' tendency to punish anyone who exercises their Sixth Amendment right to take their case to trial with a far harsher sentence than they would have received had they accepted a plea deal.

Many of the people serving life sentences for marijuana were never caught with so much as a seed or a bud—their convictions are based solely on the testimony of others trying to avoid prison time by "cooperating" with authorities. This type of testimony put Paul Free (www.FreePaulFree.com) behind bars, even though he can clearly prove, from physical evidence and from the witnesses who later recanted and claimed they were threatened to make them frame him, that he did NOT commit the marijuana crime in question. Still others like Chicago truck mechanic Craig Cesal (www.FreeCraigCesal.com) and craftsman and stay-at-home dad John Knock (JohnKnock.com) had no prior felonies on their records.

Presidential clemency remains the best hope for marijuana lifers, most of whom are now senior citizens who have already served decades behind bars, although the practice still goes on. James Romans (www.facebook.com/jimmyromanslifeforpot) received his life sentence in 2013. Sadly, most of the world has forgotten the marijuana lifers, if they ever knew they existed in the first place.

that a juror cannot be punished for his vote, regardless of his reason for voting that way.

It takes only a single person to nullify a jury and create a mistrial. The prosecution may roll the judicial dice and try the defendant again, but often they won't. If you can convince the other jurors to vote not guilty as well, the defendant will be free.

Granted, if you announce your intention to nullify the jury during the legal interview process known as *voir dire*, you will never get placed on a jury. You will need to tell the court that you have the ability to listen to the facts and make an objective decision, which is, in fact, what you should do. And if in listening to the facts you find the law corrupt, do not be afraid to vote your conscience. Learn more about your rights as a juror and how to use jury nullification to stop people from going to prison for pot from the Fully Informed Jury Association's website at www.fija.org.

◀ *Let your swag speak for you! Get this fun tote and others at Etsy.com*

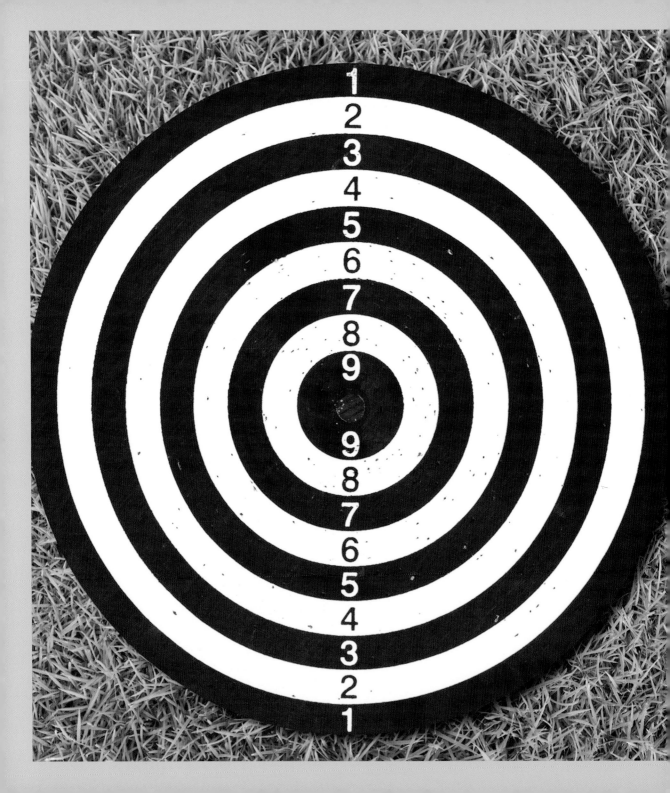

CHAPTER 17

GET ON YOUR HIGH HORSE:
how to WIN ANY ARGUMENT
about MARIJUANA

Be forewarned: If you come out of the cannabis closet and start talking honestly about your marijuana use and the need for legalization and reform, expect one of two things to happen:

1. Your listeners will want to know more and the subject may dominate the conversation from that point on. Most people's curiosity has been piqued by the extensive media coverage that cannabis has enjoyed since Colorado and Washington became the first states to legalize recreational marijuana in 2012. If you know your facts and come across as credible, people will want to learn more. Go ahead and answer their questions! Or . . .

2. Your listeners will challenge you. Don't worry; it happens far less often than you'd think, and, even if it does, relax. You've got this.

This chapter provides a credible, fact-based rebuttal for every classic prohibitionist fear, concern, or rant. Get ready to go back to high school debate club. Hopefully that won't invoke too many painful memories.

Even if you believe every shred of prohibitionist propaganda at face value, there is no credible argument on earth that can justify the expense and damage the war on cannabis has wreaked on both people around the world and our environment. Before you embark on the quest of educating the world,

SHOCKING!

Marijuana Is Safer Than . . .

By now, unless you have been living under a rock or not paying attention at all, you KNOW that by every conceivable measure, marijuana is safer than alcohol. Activists in Colorado largely credit this message with helping them to pass marijuana legalization in their state.

Mason Tvert, communications director for the Marijuana Policy Project in Colorado and one of the principal drivers behind the historic 2012 vote legalizing recreational marijuana, even cowrote a book titled *Marijuana Is Safer, So Why Are We Driving People to Drink?* (Chelsea Green Publishing, 2nd ed., 2013).

You already know that it is impossible to overdose on marijuana and die. But did you know that marijuana is actually safer than, well . . . almost everything? Including:

- **Aspirin.** Depending on the size of the person ingesting it, fewer than thirty-five aspirin tablets would constitute a fatal dose.

- **Sleeping.** According to *Time* magazine, falling out of bed kills about 600 people annually in the United States. There has never been a single death attributed to marijuana overdose.

- **Water.** In a tragic news story from 2007, twenty-eight-year-old Jennifer Strange died after drinking too much water during a radio station contest that awarded a Wii game system to the contestant who could drink the most water without going to the bathroom. The cause of death was ruled as water intoxication, a condition that occurs when a person drinks so much water that the body's nutrients become so diluted they can no longer do their jobs.

- **Food.** In 1988 Drug Enforcement Agency administrative judge Francis Young stated:

  > In strict medical terms, marijuana is far safer than many foods we commonly consume. For example, eating 10 raw potatoes can result in a toxic response. By comparison, it is physically impossible to eat enough marijuana to induce death. Marijuana in its natural form is one of the safest therapeutically active substances known to man. By any measure of rational analysis marijuana can be safely used within the supervised routine of medical care.

know in advance that credible facts and science are not enough to convince some people. Not everyone is going to stop believing the lies and start believing you. But some will. And each new person who sees the light will mean things changing for the better.

The truth is the truth, and the facts will always trump any prohibitionist argument against cannabis. So keep talking about it!

Let's say that someone is challenging you. Relax. He or she has a limited supply of anti-marijuana arguments, and you can refute each and every one of them with facts, science, and common sense. Sometimes it takes but a moment's thought to dismiss the absurdity of the argument, as in numbers 1, 3, 5, and 8, below. In other cases the truth may be obscured by biased studies and skewed statistics: See numbers 2 and 4 below. But in all cases, the facts win and prohibitionists, while entitled to their own opinions, are never entitled to their own facts.

Let's take a look at the most frequently used infamous classic prohibitionist talking points. Let the debunking begin!

UNINFORMED TALKING POINT #1:
Marijuana is a gateway to harder drugs like meth, crack, and heroin.

The truth is . . .

This lie is repeated so often and with such authority that many people, and unfortunately many so-called reporters, simply accept it at face value. The problem is there is no credible evidence to back up the claim.

Prohibitionists like to quote a National Institute on Drug Abuse study that says that a person who smokes marijuana is more than 104 times more likely to use cocaine than a person who never tries pot. But the study ignores the fact that the statistic in no way proves the cause. As University of Albany professor of psychology Mitch Earleywine eloquently puts it, "Just because something comes first doesn't

make it the cause of what comes next, as I have shown to my children countless times with a simple game of pull my finger."

Even the government's own studies don't back up the gateway drug theory. For instance, in 2009, 2.3 million people reported trying cannabis, compared with 617,000 who admitted trying cocaine and 180,000 who admitted trying heroin.

It could be argued that prohibition itself is the cause of some marijuana smokers experimenting with hard drugs. After all, if they didn't have to go to a back alley drug dealer to get marijuana, most people would never even be exposed to anything else.

The tragic thing about this particular talking point is that it keeps the public from realizing marijuana's true potential to fight harmful addictions. Science shows that cannabis can have enormous value as an exit drug, helping addicts to reduce or eliminate their intake of alcohol and other addictive substances.

A team of investigators from Canada and the United States published survey data in the journal *Addiction Research and Theory* reporting that three-quarters of medical cannabis consumers admit to using marijuana as a substitute for prescription drugs, alcohol, or some other illicit substance.

Other reports back up the claim, including a 2010 study published in the *Harm*

Reduction Journal that found cannabis-using adults enrolled in substance abuse treatment programs fared as well as or better than non-users in various categories, including completing treatment.

Marijuana can also protect against more harmful substances. A 2009 study by investigators at the University of California at San Diego reported cannabis-consuming binge drinkers experienced significantly less white matter brain damage than those who only consumed alcohol.

For years researchers and harm reduction specialists believed the value of cannabis as an exit drug came in the form of a less harmful behavioral substitution. Astounding new research suggests it's much more than that and that cannabis can actually help treat addiction at a biological level by blocking the receptors in the brain responsible for sending signals for craving.

According to Dr. Amanda Reiman, policy manager for the Drug Policy Alliance, "The palliative effects of cannabis can assist in reducing cravings and the chance of relapse while providing a safer psychoactive substitution. We're talking about a wellness model, about keeping the body in balance by introducing cannabinoids into the system instead of other substances."

UNINFORMED TALKING POINT #2:
Marijuana is addictive.

The truth is . . .

According to a National Institute of Medicine study from 1999, fewer than 10 percent of those who try marijuana ever meet the clinical criteria for dependence, whereas 32 percent of tobacco users and 15 percent of alcohol users do.

While marijuana users may develop a dependency, cannabis doesn't meet the level of a physical addiction that includes devastating withdrawal symptoms like those experienced when ceasing use of alcohol or harder drugs. In reality, a heavy cannabis consumer who stops suddenly may experience withdrawal on par with a regular coffee drinker who stops her daily caffeine habit, but many experience no withdrawal symptoms at all.

According to federal data, the number of marijuana treatment admissions referred by the criminal justice system rose from 48 percent in 1992 to 58 percent in 2006, but only 45 percent of those marijuana admissions actually met the *Diagnostic and Statistical Manual of Mental Disorders* criteria for marijuana dependence. More than a third hadn't even used marijuana at all in the entire month prior to admission for treatment. The obvious takeaway is that just because the court orders treatment, or makes it a condition of avoiding prison, does not mean the person in question is a marijuana addict. But have no doubt that each and every one of those people will be counted as an addict when the treatment centers apply for more drug war funding.

Statistically, even the number of people admitted for treatment is low compared to the number of marijuana users. According to the federal Substance Abuse and Mental Health Services Administration, in 2010 only 1.1 percent of cannabis users 12 and older sought treatment for addiction. The highest proportion of treatment admissions (14.8 percent) was in the twenty-five to twenty-nine age group.

Keep in mind over half of those admissions were compelled to seek treatment in order to avoid prison, and the actual percentage of "addicts" is less than half of that, or about 7 percent.

Even anecdotal evidence reinforces marijuana's non-addictive qualities. Think of all the people you know who used marijuana in their youth and then stopped, with no ill effect. Registered Nurse Lanny Swerdlow, who managed a California medical marijuana clinic for more than five years, says seniors made up one of the largest demographics seeking medical marijuana recommendations at his clinic. Most of them had used cannabis in their youth and stopped. When Lanny questioned why they'd stopped, they usually mentioned "career" or "family." But not a single person ever said it was because of problems they had with the substance.

UNINFORMED TALKING POINT #3:
Today's marijuana is vastly stronger and more dangerous than that of the 1960s.
The truth is . . .

It wasn't dangerous then and it isn't dangerous now. However, this talking point is partially true because, according to federal studies done in the 1980s, the THC content of U.S. marijuana averaged around 3 percent. Current testing does show an increase to an average of 5.6 percent THC by 2009.

However, the range of what was available then and now remains virtually unchanged. Stronger weed existed in the past—the range of THC samples shows that it did—but the lab-tested samples we have from back then are extremely limited in variety and scope.

So, the validity of this claim depends on what you were smoking back in the 1960s. There was good stuff back then, just as there is now. If you're old enough and were lucky enough to get your hands on some in the 1960s, you'll remember Thai Sticks, Panama Red, or Maui Wowie, all as potent as today's strains. However, with the legalization of medical and even recreational marijuana, there is a WHOLE lot more of the good stuff around these days. If you live in a legal or medicinally legal state, gone are the days of smoking schwag and brick weed.

The statement also ignores the fact that studies show marijuana smokers naturally adjust to the level of potency. "When the potency is stronger, the user tends to smoke less," says Dr. Mitch Earleywine.

So, in the ultimate ironic pro-marijuana talking point, it could be argued that stronger marijuana could actually result in individuals smoking less cannabis overall!

It's all much ado about nothing. Even if you take the claims at face value, increased potency does not make marijuana harmful, as we learned in Chapter 3. Nor it does it change the plant's characteristics and magically transform it into a "dangerous" and/or

"addictive" substance. Regardless of potency, THC is nontoxic to healthy cells or organs and cannot cause a fatal overdose.

To further underline the hypocrisy of this ridiculous prohibitionist fear-mongering, consider the fact that any doctor can legally, without any issue in any state, prescribe the pharmaceutical Marinol, which is 100 percent THC, and, unlike the natural plant, comes with a host of serious side effects. For the record, Marinol is a Schedule III drug, while the natural plant remains a Schedule I with "no acceptable medical use" at the federal level. It is also far more expensive than top-shelf marijuana from a dispensary.

UNINFORMED TALKING POINT #4:
We already have enough problems with alcohol, so why add another legal addiction?

The truth is . . .

First of all, see Talking Point #2 above and debunk the "Marijuana is addictive" argument. Continue with the fact that comparing marijuana to alcohol is like comparing apples to orangutans, and watch this argument fall apart fast. By every conceivable measure, marijuana is safer than alcohol and does not cause anywhere near the harms and expense on society that alcohol does. So, if prohibitionists really wanted to protect society, they

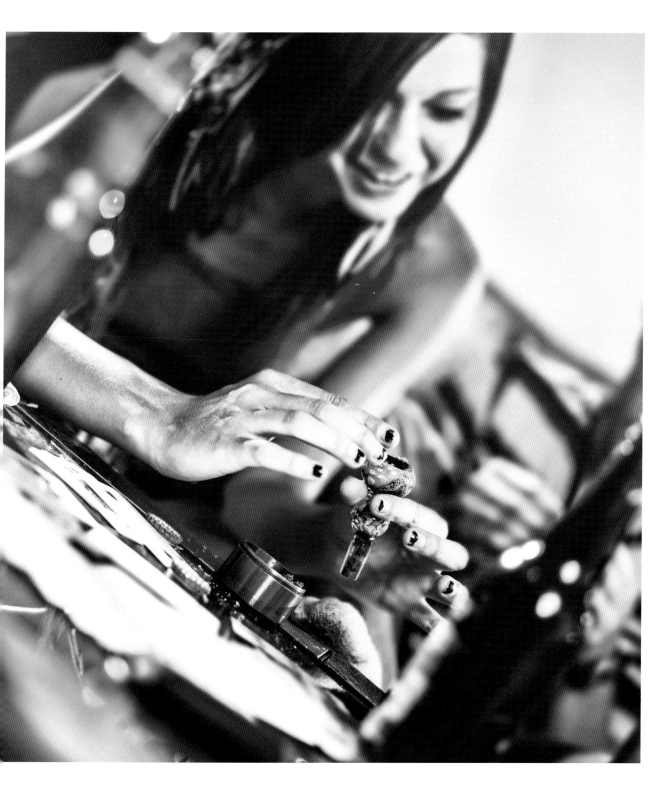

would encourage responsible adults to relax with marijuana instead of alcohol, instead of trying to ban it.

A quick look at the facts shows there is no logical reason to treat these substances as even close to equal, so let's stop doing so.

Alcohol: A 2011 analysis published in the *American Journal of Preventive Medicine* concluded that an estimated 80,000 lives are lost annually due to either excessive drinking or accidental death by overdose in the United States alone. A February 2011 World Health Organization report says that alcohol consumption is responsible for 4 percent of all deaths worldwide.

Marijuana: There has never been a single death credibly attributed to marijuana use, and it is in fact impossible to fatally overdose on marijuana.

Alcohol: According to a 2009 report in the *British Columbia Mental Health and Addictions Journal*, the annual health-related cost of alcohol consumption is $165 per user.

Marijuana: The same report puts the health-related costs of marijuana use at $20 per user.

Alcohol: Science has proven beyond a doubt that excessive alcohol use damages brain cells.

Marijuana: Unlike alcohol, cannabis is a neuroprotectant, meaning that it does not damage brain cells but actually

helps to protect them. A 2009 University of California at San Diego study that focused on binge drinkers showed that those who had also used cannabis experienced less brain damage than those who used alcohol alone.

Alcohol: Withdrawal from heavy alcohol use is a potentially life-threatening process that comes with serious detox symptoms, including tremors, vomiting, severe anxiety, seizures, and, in extreme cases, delirium tremens (also called DTs), which manifest as confusion, rapid heartbeat, and fever.

SHOCKING!
Your Tax Dollars Wasted . . . Again

Decades of studies have failed to show a link between marijuana use and violent behavior, but that has not stopped the U.S. government, in its infinite fiscal wisdom, from spending your tax dollars trying to create one.

The National Institute on Drug Abuse, which as you recall will ONLY fund studies looking for negative consequences of marijuana use, granted $1.86 million to the University of Buffalo's Research Institute on Addictions to investigate the alleged link between marijuana use and aggression. The study will run from 2013 to 2017 and will follow couples in which one or both partners use marijuana to determine whether its use "results in affective, cognitive, or behavioral effects consistent with partner aggression."

Marijuana: Withdrawal from marijuana use is equivalent to a caffeine addict giving up coffee; in many instances, there are no symptoms.

Alcohol: Alcohol use is associated with a cornucopia of cancers, including lung, esophagus, stomach, colon, liver, and prostate, among others.

Marijuana: No credible study has linked marijuana use to cancer risk. In fact, a number of studies show marijuana can protect against cancer and actually kill cancer cells, even in long-term marijuana users (see Chapter 6).

Alcohol: The National Highway Traffic Safety Administration reported in 2013 that 28 people die each day in the United States as a result of drunk driving.

Marijuana: As surprising as it may sound, scientific data actually show that traffic fatalities go down in states that have enacted medical marijuana laws (see Talking Point #7 below).

Alcohol: Study after study confirms a link between alcohol consumption and an increase in aggressive and violent behavior. According to the National Institute on Alcohol Abuse and Alcoholism, more than a quarter of all violent crimes—and a full three-quarters of all incidents of intimate partner violence—are committed by someone who had recently been drinking.

Marijuana: Numerous studies as far back as those commissioned by Richard Nixon and as recent as 2010 show no link between marijuana use and violence. Poll any beat cop on how many domestic violence calls they answer attributed only to marijuana use, and the answer is invariably zero.

UNINFORMED TALKING POINT #5:
Marijuana makes you lazy, fat, and unmotivated.

The truth is . . .

Oh, really? Tell that to John F. Kennedy, Jimmy Carter, George H. W. Bush, Bill Clinton, Barack Obama, Maya Angelou, Bill Gates, Carl Sagan, Jay-Z, Michael Phelps, Sir Richard Branson, Ted Turner, Jennifer Aniston, Jon Stewart, Cameron Diaz, Sarah Palin, Bill Maher, Willie Nelson, Merle Haggard, Rihanna, Miley Cyrus, Kirstin Dunst, Morgan Freeman, Oliver Stone, Madonna, Susan Sarandon, Frances McDormand, Martha Stewart, and countless other overachieving marijuana users and former marijuana users.

Even Cheech and Chong, the two people on earth most responsible for this absurd stereotype, are in actuality successful entertainment industry icons with careers that have spanned more than four decades and are still going strong. Not too shabby for a couple of slacker stoners.

As to the fat part, a study published in the *American Journal of Epidemiology* showed that obesity rates for marijuana users were about a third less than those of their abstaining counterparts, even when taking external factors into account and despite marijuana's ability to induce the munchies.

If you are lazy and unmotivated without weed, you will continue to be lazy and unmotivated with it. And if you're not, you won't. 'Nuff said. This argument is too silly to merit any kind of serious debate.

use had no negative effect on cognitive function or long-term memory.

Additionally, cannabis's role as a neuroprotectant has been shown to prevent brain cell damage in binge drinkers and may prevent diseases like Alzheimer's that diminish mental capacity.

Finally, to make a prohibitionist's head explode, don't forget to cite U.S. patent number 6,630,507, held by the U.S. government on cannabinoids as antioxidants and neuroprotectants (see Chapter 6). How can marijuana kill brain cells when the federal government owns a patent saying it protects them?

UNINFORMED TALKING POINT #6:
Marijuana kills brain cells and makes you stupid.

Short-term memory loss is one of the few actual marijuana side effects, but it only lasts for the duration of the high.

Researchers at the University of Melbourne and the Australian National University's Center for Mental Health Research published a 2011 study that looked at the impact of cannabis use on various measures of memory and intelligence in over 2,000 self-identified marijuana consumers and nonusers over an eight-year period. They found that even long-term heavy marijuana

UNINFORMED TALKING POINT #7:
Legalizing marijuana will cause more deaths and accidents on the highway because of all the stoned drivers.

The truth is . . .

There are already thousands of marijuana drivers on the highway and it hasn't resulted in the bloodbath of carnage the fear-mongering prohibitionists predicted when states first started legalizing medical marijuana.

It is true that in some doses and in some people, marijuana affects perception and psychomotor performance. However, studies also show that, unlike alcohol, which increases risky behavior, marijuana tends to make people more cautious. Cannabis users studied seemed aware of their impairment and compensated for it. Furthermore, long-term users build up a tolerance that can eliminate impairment entirely.

Surveys of marijuana-related traffic fatalities almost always show that alcohol was also involved.

In one of the most counterintuitive facts about marijuana—so much so that a lot of people are not going to believe you—University of Colorado at Denver professor Daniel Rees and Montana State University professor D. Mark Anderson concluded in 2012 that traffic fatalities actually decreased by 9 percent in states that have legalized medical marijuana. The exact reason for this is still under debate, but popular wisdom correlates increased marijuana use with decreased alcohol use, and alcohol use, by every objective barometer, causes far more devastation on the roads.

The prohibitionist spin in states like Washington that impose mandatory per se driving limits is that police have arrested thousands of stoned drivers. These laws state that if a driver tests positive for having X amount of THC in his system (5 nanograms in Washington), he is considered to be under the influence. But because marijuana stays in the system for over six weeks, the presence of cannabis in the body has no correlation with impairment levels. Furthermore, studies show that marijuana produces little or no vehicle-handling impairment, and overall rates of highway accidents appear not to be significantly affected by marijuana's more widespread use.

UNINFORMED TALKING POINT #8:
Legalizing marijuana will make it more available to kids.

Prohibitionists like to trot out this errant point often, so be prepared.

The truth is . . .

Back alley drug dealers do not ask for ID, but legal marijuana dispensaries do. If you really want to keep marijuana from kids, regulate it. As it currently stands, a kid can get weed far more easily than she can get alcohol. Why? Because of regulations that impose serious consequences on liquor stores that sell to kids.

This fact alone should be enough to put an end to the argument, but some people are extreme idiots. For them, point out studies like the ones conducted by Dr. Esther Choo at Brown University (2009) or Dr. Mitch Earleywine at the University of Albany (2005) that show either no change in teen use after legalization, or a decrease.

UNINFORMED TALKING POINT #9:
Marijuana smoke causes lung cancer and is as or more dangerous than tobacco smoke.

The truth is . . .

A study at UCLA, much to lead researcher Dr. Donald Tashkin's surprise, showed that cannabis smoke does not cause lung cancer, and in fact could very well protect against it. In 2012, presenters at the annual meeting of the American Academy for Cancer Research reported that subjects who regularly inhale cannabis smoke are at no greater risk of lung cancer than those who consume it occasionally or not at all. After examining 6 case-control studies conducted between 1999 and 2012 and involving over 5,000 subjects (2,159 cases and 2,985 controls) from around the world, the presenters stated, "Our pooled results showed no significant association between the intensity, duration, or cumulative consumption of cannabis smoke and the risk of lung cancer overall or in never smokers."

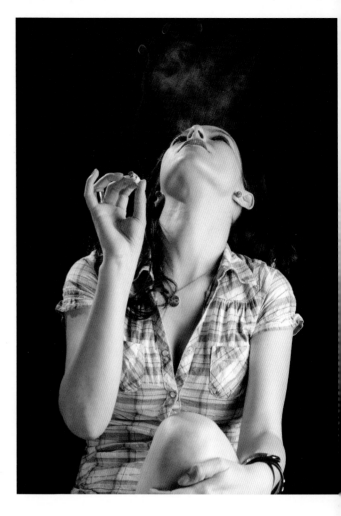

HOW TO:

Evaluate the Credibility and Importance of Any Study

Every now and again a study comes on the scene that touts a negative effect of cannabis, and the mainstream media never refrains from jumping on it, even if only a handful of subjects were involved and the results are tenuous at best. Before you get all up in arms about the potential harms, check out the study itself and consider the points below. I've yet to find one that holds up under scrutiny. Likewise, you should turn the same critical eye toward pro-marijuana studies. Not that I have any doubt about marijuana's miraculous healing potential, but, as the industry grows, the charlatans and hucksters out for nothing more than a quick buck will also become more common. Be sure the study you are looking at, positive or negative, merits the weight you give it.

Consider these points:

- How many subjects were studied and over what period of time? More subjects over a longer duration give more credibility to the study's results.

- Was the study conducted on humans or animals? I am not saying that animal studies have no merit, but a long-term study on a large number of human subjects would mean more, assuming it was properly conducted and evaluated.

- If applicable, was it a blind or double-blind study?

- Who funded the study, and do they stand to gain by the study's results? A study claiming that marijuana is addictive sponsored by an association of rehab counselors and clinics offers less credibility that one paid for by a more neutral entity.

- Did the study take tobacco use, prescription and/or illegal drug use, lifestyle, or other external factors into consideration? A lot of "marijuana as a gateway drug" theories and studies fail to do so. But if these influencing factors are not accounted for, you can't credibly attribute the study results to cannabis use.

- Do the numbers actually mean what is implied? For instance, prohibitionists like to quote the huge numbers of people who seek treatment for marijuana "addictions." What they fail to mention is that the vast majority of those enrolled in treatment programs are not there because of need, but rather as a condition of avoiding prison. As long as people are forced into treatment, those stats are meaningless. You'll find a similar situation when looking more closely at marijuana-related emergency room visits.

- If a study started out looking for a negative, and in fact found a positive—like Dr. Donald Tashkin's study at UCLA, mentioned above, that showed that smoking marijuana does NOT contribute to lung cancer—or vice versa, give it extra credibility. If said study's sponsor immediately cuts its funding upon knowledge of the unexpected results, chances are even greater the study was on to something big and somebody stands to lose a lot of money if it is discovered.

THROUGH *the* YEARS *with* MARY JANE: A CANNABIS CHRONOLOGY

🌿 **CIRCA 2,700 BC** First recorded use of cannabis as medicine by Emperor Shen Neng, aka "The Father of Chinese Medicine."

🌿 **1213 BC** Cannabis pollen found on the mummy of Ramesses II.

🌿 **10TH CENTURY AD** First documented case of "Reefer Madness" when Arab physician Ibn Wahshiyah claims the "odor of hashish is lethal."

🌿 **1538** CE William Turner, considered the first English botanist, writes of marijuana's medical merits.

🌿 **1839–1841** William O'Shaughnessy presents cannabis research to the Medical and Physical Society of Calcutta and brings quantities of cannabis and hemp to the Royal Botanical Gardens at Kew and the British Pharmaceutical Society, thus lunching the dawn of modern medical marijuana.

🌿 **1890** Sir John Russell Reynolds, Queen Victoria's personal physician for thirty-seven years, writes of the many healing and therapeutic properties of cannabis. While we don't know for sure if the queen partook, it is quite likely her doctor, who regularly prescribed marijuana for a variety of reasons, did advise it.

🌿 **1914** El Paso, Texas, passes America's first anti-marijuana ordinance after a Mexican immigrant, supposedly high on "marihuana" (which most people did not realize was the same cannabis that was in their medicine cabinets), went crazy and shot up the town.

🌿 **1930** The Federal Bureau of Narcotics is formed. Director Harry Anslinger's racist anti-weed agenda would wreak havoc through five presidential administrations until he finally left the office in 1962 and took his crusade global, serving for two years as the United States' representative to the United Nations Narcotics Commission.

🌿 **1937** Congress passes the Marijuana Tax Act, which places an onerous tax on marijuana and hemp and imposes fines and prison time on those who don't comply. The legislation effectively outlawed cannabis and hemp while circumventing Constitutional restrictions.

🌿 **1938** *Popular Mechanics* claims that more than 25,000 products could be made from hemp—everything from cellophane to dynamite.

🌿 **1944** Despite its illegal status, the government gives farmers free seeds, and more than 375,000 acres of hemp are harvested in part of the "Hemp for Victory" campaign to provide necessary supplies for the war effort.

🌿 **1944** At the behest of New York City Mayor Fiorello La Guardia, the New York Academy of Medicine publishes the results of an extensive, well-researched, six-year study confirming that, contrary to popular belief, marijuana use does not induce violence, insanity, or sex crimes.

🌿 **1952** The Boggs Act implements harsher punishments and mandatory minimum sentences for drug-related offenses. A first-time marijuana possession offense carries a 2–10-year minimum sentence and a fine of up to $20,000.

🌿 **1960s** Marijuana popularity enjoys a huge resurgence thanks to the hippies and the anti–Vietnam War movement.

🌿 **1961** Harry Anslinger persuades the United Nations to convince more than 100 countries to unify their various drug agreements into a single inflexible convention that essentially makes marijuana illegal around the world. This agreement still stands, keeping countries locked into a destructive policy through the threat of possible sanctions and making for sticky legal situations when these countries want to move beyond the prohibitionist mindset.

🌿 **1969** Anthropologist Margaret Mead testifies before Congress in favor of legalizing marijuana. Congress keeps marijuana illegal.

🌿 **1969** Timothy Leary challenges the constitutionality of the Marijuana Stamp Tax Act in front of the Supreme Court, arguing that the law violates the Fifth Amendment as it requires those paying the tax to incriminate themselves. The court unanimously agrees.

🌿 **1970** In response to Leary's Supreme Court victory, Congress passes The Controlled Substances Act, which labels marijuana a Schedule I drug, the same category as heroin.

🌿 **1972** Richard Nixon coins the phrase "War on Drugs" after discrediting the scientifically researched findings of his own commission, which recommended Congress and state legislatures decriminalize the use and casual distribution of marijuana for personal use. The commission's findings further stated that "neither the marihuana user nor the drug itself can be said to constitute a danger to public safety."

🌿 **1973** Dr. Tod Mikuriya reprints William O'Shaugnessey's Calcutta paper as the lead article in *Marijuana: Medical Papers 1839–1972*, sparking new interest in medical marijuana and prompting hundreds more articles and studies on the benefits of cannabis therapy.

🌿 **1973** Oregon becomes the first state to completely decriminalize marijuana.

🌿 **1979** Former Canadian First Lady Margaret Trudeau reveals in her book *Beyond Reason* that she "smoked pot with the best of them and came to love it."

🍃 **1989** President George HW Bush declares an all-new "War on Drugs" in a televised speech and creates the largest increase in drug-war funding in history, to the tune of $2.2 billion.

🍃 **1996** California legalizes medical marijuana.

🍃 **2005** In her holiday message, sent while she was incarcerated in federal prison, Martha Stewart writes: "I beseech you all to think about these women—to encourage the American people to ask for reforms, both in sentencing guidelines, in length of incarceration for nonviolent first-time offenders, and for those involved in drug-taking."

🍃 **2006** Fulla Nayak, believed to be the world's oldest woman, passes away in India at the age of 125. Nayak credited her longevity to her daily marijuana smoking habit.

🍃 **2009** Former Miss New Jersey Georgine DiMaria publicly advocates for medical marijuana, admitting she personally finds it helpful, paving the way for other contestants to get green. In 2001, Miss California Alyssa Campanella went on to take the Miss USA crown with her pro–medical marijuana response to a pageant-interview question.

🍃 **2012** Colorado and Washington legalize recreational marijuana.

🍃 **2012** Uruguay becomes the first nation to legalize recreational marijuana.

🍃 **2014** Sarah Silverman announces to the world from the Red Carpet at the Emmy Awards that she is carrying "liquid pot" in her purse.

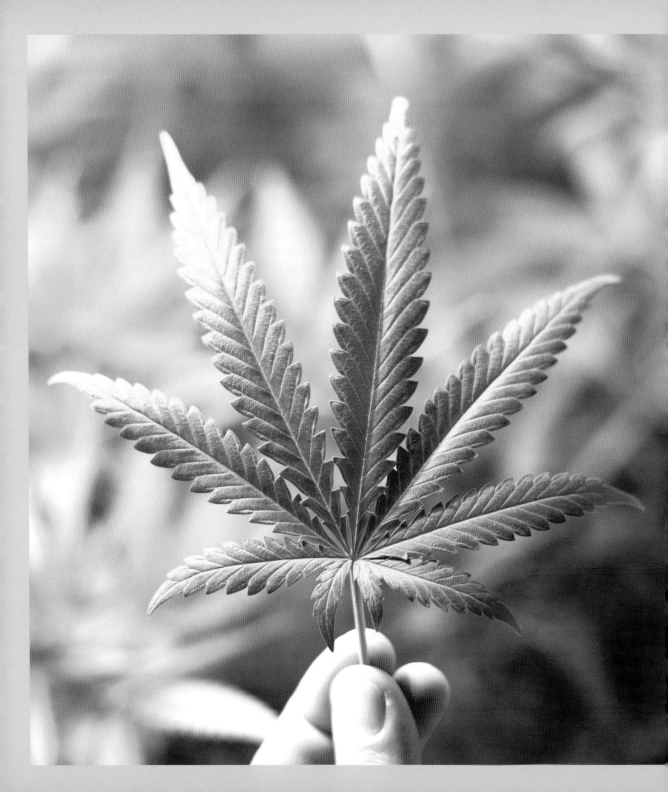

ACKNOWLEDGMENTS

Thank you to all these wonderful people who either helped with this book and/or put up with me and gave me support while I wrote it:

Mitch Mandell (as always); my editor Laura Mazer and all the fine folks at Seal Press, as well as Rachel Sarah; my agents Janet Rosen and Sheree Bykofsky; Dale Gieringer, Kandice Hawes-Lopez, Amy Povah, Ellen Komp, Sabrina Fendrick, Diane Goldstein, Stephen Downing, Paul Armentano, Dr. Jeffrey Raber, Dr. Amanda Reiman, Dr. Mitch Earleywine, Dr. Lakisha Jenkins, Dr. Richard Palmquist, Dr. Robert Melamede, Michael Levinsohn, Jennifer Ani, Allison Margolin, Alexis Wilson Briggs, Lauren Vazquez, Jeff Spellerberg, Wanda Smith, Catrina Coleman, Joe Grumbine, Liz Grumbine, Stephanie Landa, Kathie Zamanjahromi, Chris Brown, April Price, Chuck Burnes, Bambi Burnes, Richard Burnes, Tracy Burnes, Cynthia Johnston, Veridiana Noriega, Jessica Lux, Bill Levers, Jeff Levers, Liz McDuffie, Steve Elliott, Dale Sky Jones, Pebbles Trippet, Debby Goldsberry, Jared Allaway, Madeline Martinez and the Martinez Family, Diane Fornbacher, Angela Bacca, Vanessa Waltz, Beth Curtis, Charlie Bott, Erin Purchase, Brandon Krenzler, Mykayla Comstock, Dan Rush, Lindsey Rinehart, Candace Junkin, Deanna Jean Ryther, Mickey Martin, Robert Brown, January Thomas, Barb Brisson; Cannabis POWs Paul Free, Randy Lanier, Craig Cesal, James Romans, and Larry Duke (all five serving LIFE WITHOUT PAROLE for nonviolent marijuana offenses), Dustin Costa, Marilyn Greene, Gerry Campbell, Luke Scarmazzo, Weldon Angelos, John Marcinkewciz, and Christopher Williams.

And a special thank you to Lanny Swerdlow. It may seem strange to dedicate a book for women to a man, but Lanny is well in touch with his feminine side and I don't think he would mind. Plus, he is the person who inspired me to become a cannabis activist. So it's only fitting that a book dedicated to furthering his message be dedicated to him. Thank you, Lanny, I am forever grateful to you for the profoundly rewarding way in which you changed my life.

INDEX

A

a/k/a Tommy Chong, 151
AARP magazine, 147
aches and pains, 67
ACLU Criminal Law Reform
    Project, 193
Activated Carbon Fiber bags, 46
Adams, Ryan, 165
Addiction Research and
    Theory, 201
addiction, studies on, 202–203
Adlon, Pamela, 152
"Adopt a Prisoner" program, 194
advocacy actions, 189–197
aeroponic system, 80
Aerosmith, 167
affirmative defense, 88
Afroman, 165
aggression, studies on, 206
airport security, 55
alcohol, 68, 204, 206–207
Alice in Wonderland, 149
Allaway, Jared, 195
Allen, Woody, 155
Ambrose, Lauren, 154
American Academy for Cancer
    Research, 210
American Civil Liberties
    Union (ACLU), 54

American Drug War: The Last
    White Hope, 151
American Drug War 2:
    Cannabis Destiny, 151
American Herbalist Guild, 131
American Journal of
    Epidemiology, 62, 208
American Journal of
    Preventive Medicine, 206
American Medical Association
    (AMA), 57
American Thyroid
    Association, 63
Amsterdam, Netherlands, 169–171
An Unmarried Woman, 143–144
Anderson, Mark, 209
Angelou, Maya, 207
Ani, Jen, 130
Aniston, Jennifer, 2, 155, 207
Ann Arbor Hash Bash, 176
Annie Hall, 144
Anslinger, Harry, 57, 213, 214
arrest, consequences of, 49–50
asthma, 68

B

Baker, George, 161
Balk, Fairuza, 146
balloon style vapes, 27–28

bargain shopping, 23
Barr, Roseanne, 155
Barrymore, Drew, 147
"Because I Got High," 165
Being John Malkovich, 144
Beyond Reason, 214
Bhang Lassi, 123
Big Book of Buds, 12
Big C, The (Showtime), 154
Black Sabbath, 161
Block, Robert, 122
"Blueberry Yum Yum," 159
blunt, 19
Blunt, James, 167
Bob & Ted & Carol & Alice, 143
body weight, 73
Bogarting, 25
Boggs Act, 213
bongs, 21, 23, 141
border guards, 55
Boston Freedom Rally, 176, 178
Branson, Richard, 207
Breakfast at Tiffany's, 144
Brewer & Shipley, 159
British Columbia Mental
    Health and Addictions
    Journal, 206
British Pharmaceutical Society,
    212

British Royal National Hospital for Rheumatic Disease, 63
bronchial conditions, 68
Bronner, Emanuel, 76
bubble hash, 34
bubbler pipe, 23
buds, 12
budtender, 46
Buford, Mojo, 164
Bull Durham, 144
Bureau of Narcotics, 57
"Burn One Down," 158
Burnett, Carol, 154
Bush, George H. W., 207, 215
butane hash oil (BHO), 34
butter and oil recipe, 106–107
buying options, 5–10, 12

C
C&C Music Factory, 167
California Department of Social Services (CDSS), 186
California Medical Marijuana Program, 186
California, State of, 131
Californication (Showtime), 152
Calloway, Cab, and His Cotton Club Orchestra, 155
Campanella, Alyssa, 215
"Can Anybody Hear Me?," 158
cancer, 60, 62
Cancer Prevention Research, 60

cannabidiol (CBD), 66
cannabinoids, 8
Cannabis Café, 179
Cannabis Indica, 6–7
Cannabis Sativa, 6, 7
Cannabist, The, 147
cannaigrette dressing, 114
Canned Heat, 164
Cannon, Dyan, 143
car searches, 54, 55–56
carburetor, 21
careers, 181–187
Carlin, George, 155
Carter, Jimmy, 207
cashed, 25
Cesal, Craig, 197
challenges, and rebuttals, 199–211
"Champagne and Reefer," 164
Charlie and the Chocolate Factory, 149
checkpoint traps, 54
Cheech and/or Chong, 1, 151, 207
Cheese, Richard, 162
cherry, 19
Child Protective Services (CPS), 95, 130, 131, 194
Children, 125–131
conversations with, 126–128
and law enforcement, 95, 130
legalization and, 209
medical marijuana for, 128–129, 131
Chitty Chitty Bang Bang, 149
Choo, Esther, 209

chronology, cannabis, 212–215
Church, Eric, 165
Clinton, Bill, 207
clones, 79–80
collectives, 43
Colorado, marijuana in, 178–179
Commander Cody and His Lost Planet Airmen, 161
concentrates, 31–37, 109–111
Conroy, Frances, 146, 154
consent, searches and, 52
Controlled Substances Act, 214
cooking, cannabis and, 97–115
buds, 108–109
concentrates, 109–111
dosage and, 102–104
draining and straining, 107–108
fat and, 103
preparation and, 102
recipes, 77, 106–107, 114–115, 123, 134
temperature, 104
versus inhaling, 97–99
cooperatives, 43
cops, undercover, 41
Cosby, Bill, 155
cost, of marijuana, 47
cotton mouth, 121
Country Joe and the Fish, 161
cramping, 67
criminal marijuana sentencing, 197
critical extraction oils, 34
cultural differences, 191

Culture magazine, 147
curing, 94–95
custody battles, 130
cuttings, 79–80
Cypress Hill, 159
Cyrus, Miley, 166, 207

D
dabbing, 34–35, 37
Dale, Dick, 159
dank, 7
dank chocolate espresso
    brownies, 115
"Dark Sunglasses," 165
Department of Health and
    Human Services, 64
dependency, 202–203
designer joints, 137
detention, involuntary, 52–53
detention, police, 52–53
DeWitt, Rosemarie, 152
diabetes, 62
*Diagnostic and Statistical
    Manual of Mental
    Disorders*, 202
Diaz, Cameron, 144, 147, 207
"Dieman Noba Smoke Tafee,"
    163
Diff'rent Strokes, 151
Dillard, Hartford, and Dillard,
    159
DiMaria, Georgine, 215
dispensaries, 43–48
"Do You Dig My Jive?," 156
documentary movies, 150–151

"Don't Bogart Me," 163
"Don't Step on the Grass,
    Sam," 156, 158
doobie, 18
dosing, 98, 99
"Down to Seeds and Stems
    Again Blues," 161
Dr. Bronner's Magic Soaps, 76
draining, cooking and, 107–108
Dreher, Melanie, 66
driving, 46, 54, 55–56, 208–209
Drug and Alcohol Dependence,
    72
drug dependence, 68
Drug Policy Alliance (DPA),
    179, 195
duff, 28
dugout, 23
Dunst, Kirstin, 147, 207
dutchie, 19
Dylan, Bob, 161

E
ear wax, 34
Earlywine, Mitch, 201, 204, 209
Ebers Papyrus, 68
edibles, 98
Education Program for
    Licensees and
    Administrators of State-
    Licensed Residential
    Care Facilities, 186
Edwards, Ezekiel, 193
"Electric Avenue," 164
Emerald Cup, 176

emphysema, 68
entertaining, 133, 135–136
environmental issues, 82
Etheridge, Melissa, 2, 166
etiquette, smoking, 25
evidence planting, 52
exercise, 72
exit drug, 201–202
expense
    growing and, 82, 84, 85
    marijuana and, 47
expos and festivals, 172, 175–
    176, 178
extracts, 31–37
Eyes Wide Shut, 150

F
failure to protect/supervise,
    130
Falco, Edie, 154
"Family Tradition," 164
fan leaves, 12
Farrell, Gail, 159
fatty, 18
Federal Bureau of Narcotics,
    213
feminized seeds, 80
festivals, 172, 175–176, 178
fibromyalgia, 63
Fifth Dimension, The, 161
Fiji, Charlotte, 128, 154
Filthy Fregs, 162
"Fire Burns for Freedom, A,"
    158
Fish Fry Bingo, 162

flowers, 12, 80

flush, 80

"Follow Your Arrow," 165

Fonda, Jane, 144, 146

Foria, 77

Fornbacher, Diane, 125–126

Fountains of Wayne, 163

420 documentary, 150

420 games, 156, 179

420 holiday, 178

Fraternity of Man, 163

Free, Paul, 197

Freeman, Morgan, 207

fruit and vegetable pipes, 139, 141

full melt hash, 34

Fully Informed Jury Association, 197

G

ganjanduja hot chocolate, 77

gastrointestinal disorders, relief from, 67

Gates, Bill, 207

generation gaps, 190–191

Gieringer, Dale, 170

glass pipes, 19

gloves, 93

Goldberg, Whoopi, 147

GQ magazine, 147

"Granny Wontcha Smoke Some Marijuana?," 162

Grant, Eddy, 164

Grass, 151

Grateful Dead, 159

gravity bongs, 141

gravy separator, 107

Gray, Macy, 162

Griffiths, Rachel, 154

grinders, 18

grow tents, 85

growing marijuana, 79–95

    curing, 94–95

    decisions before, 80, 82

    harvesting, 90

    indoors, 83–85

    outdoors, 82–83

    plant gender, 85, 87

    security, 88–89

    terms, 79–80

    trimming, 90, 93–94

    troubleshooting, 87

Guerrero, Lalo, 156

guns, 95

Gupta, Sanjay, 60, 128, 154

Guy, Buddy "Motherfucker," 164

gynecology, 62–63

H

Haggard, Merle, 207

Hamilton Beach "Stay and Go" cookers, 105

hard drugs, marijuana as gateway to, 201

Harm Reduction Journal, 201–202

Harper, Ben, 158

Hartford, John, 162

harvests, 82–83, 87, 90

hash, 32

"Hash Pipe," 165

Hawaii Five-o (CBS), 154

headaches, relief from, 67

health, 71–77

Hearst, William Randolph, 57

heat, THC and, 9

hemp, 7

Hemp and Cannabis Foundation, 176

"Hemp for Victory" campaign, 213

"Henry," 161

Hepburn, Audrey, 144

hermaphrodites, 87

Hester, Clinton, 57

"(Hey Uncle Sam) Leave Us Pot Smokers Alone," 158

"High," 167

High Times, 147, 175, 178

High Times Cannabis Cups, 35, 175, 178

Holi Festival, 172

home searches, 56

home-testing kits, 10

honey oil, 34

hookah, 23

hookup person (HP), 39–41

hotbox, 19

household hints, 133–141

Human Solution, the (THS), 194

Humboldt County, 146

"Hush Hush," 165

hybrids, 6–7

hydroponic system, 80
Hynde, Chrissie, 158, 165, 166

I

"I Like Marijuana," 161
I Love You, Alice B. Toklas, 143
immigration points, 55
India, marijuana in, 172
indoor growing, 83–85
inflammation, relief from, 67
inhaling, 15–28
Ink Spots, 156
insomnia, relief from, 67
intelligence, studies on, 208
intercepting, 25

J

Jackson 5, 161
James, Rick, 165, 167
Jay-Z, 207
Jenkins, Lakisha, 131
jeweler's loupe, 89
Joan and Melissa: Joan Knows Best?, 155
"John Sinclair," 158
joints, 15–19
    rolling, 16, *17*
joints, designer, 137
Jones, Dale Sky, 186
Journal of Natural Products, 67
Journal of Toxicology, 9
jury duty, 195–197
Justified (FX), 152

K

Kaiser Permanente Center, 24
"Kaya," 164
Keaton, Diane, 144
Keener, Catherine, 144, 146
Keith, Toby, 159
Kennedy, John F., 207
Kenzler, Brandon, 128–129, 131
Kid Cudi, 165
kid movies, 149
kief, 28, 32
Knock, John, 197
Kottonmouth Kings, 158
Kunis, Mila, 154
Kushman, Kyle, 10

L

La Guardia, Fiorello, 213
lab tests, 8–9
labeling, law enforcement and, 88
labels, lab testing and, 8–9
labor, growing and, 82, 84
Lady Gaga, 166
Ladybud, 125
Lambert, Miranda, 165
latex gloves, 93
Laurel Canyon, 146
law enforcement, 49–57
    and children, 95, 130
    labeling and, 88
    undercover cops, 41
Law Enforcement Against Prohibition (LEAP), 56, 195
Leary, Timothy, 214

leaves, 12
Led Zeppelin, 159
Lee, Julia, and Her Boy Friends, 156
Lee, Richard, 185
legal rights, 49–57
"Legalise Me," 158
"Legalize It," 158
Lennon, John, 158
Levinsohn, Michael, 53, 56
"Light Up or Leave Me Alone," 163
lighting, growing and, 84, 85, 87
Linney, Laura, 154
Little Beach, Maui, 172
Little Feat, 164
"Little Green Bag," 161
"Live High," 163
Live magazine, 147
Lively, Blake, 146
Looney Tunes, 146
"Louie Louie," 162
Ludacris, 159
lung cancer, 27, 210
Lyme disease, 68

M

macaroni and cheese, 114–115
McDormand, Frances, 146, 147, 207
McElhone, Natascha, 152
Mad Men (AMC), 152
Madonna, 207
Maher, Bill, 207
Mamas and Papas, 156

Manhattan Transfer, 156
Maraniss, David, 25
March of the Penguins, 150
Marijuana: Medical Paers 1839-1972, 214
"Marijuana" (Country Joe and The Fish), 161
"Marijuana" (Kid Cudi), 165
"Marijuana Boogie," 156
marijuana cigarettes, 15–19
terms for, 18–19
Marijuana Is Safer, So Why Are We Driving Peiple to Drink?, 200
marijuana leaf chart, 140
Marijuana Policy Project (MPP), 147, 195, 200
marijuana, safeness of, 5, 200
Marijuana Stamp Tax Act, 57, 213, 214
Marin County, California, 130
Marinol, 204
Marley, Bob, 164
Marley, Rita, 164
Marley, Ziggy, 158
Marquez, Vanessa, 164
Martindale, Margo, 152
"Mary Jane," 165, 167
maternity, 64, 66
math conversions, 171
Matthews, Dave, 159
Maui Wowie, 203
Mazursky, Paul, 143
Mead, Margaret, 214
Mechoulam, Raphael, 8

media, letters to, 193
medibles, 98
Medical and Physical Society of Calcutta, 212
Medical Cannabis Caregivers Institute (MCC), 186
medical marijuana, 59–69
children and, 128–129, 131
state reciprocity and, 170
Melamede, Robert, 71
memory, studies on, 208
metabolism, 98
metal pipes, 19
Methicillin-resistant Staphylococcus aureus (MRSA), 67
Midler, Bette, 146, 156
Mighty Diamonds, The, 163
migraines, 67
Mikuriya, Tod, 214
Miranda warning, 53
Monroe, Ashley, 118, 165, 167
Monroe Street Fair, 176
Montana State University, study at, 204
Moody Blues, 159
Morissette, Alanis, 166
Moss, Elisabeth, 153
mother plant, 80
motivation, 207–208
Moulin Rouge, 149–150
movies, marijuana in, 143–144, 146, 147, 149–151
Mraz, Jason, 163
Multi-Disciplinary Association

for Psychedelic Studies (MAPS), 24
"munchies, the," 73
Munson, Albert, 62
Musgraves, Kacey, 165
music libraries, 158
music, marijuana in, 154–167
cannabis protest songs, 156, 158–159
celebration of, 161–163
dry periods, 159, 161
love and lust, 165, 167
oldies, 155–156
passing the joint, 163–164
stoned songs, 159
tough times and, 164–165
Musical Youth, 25, 163

N

names, marijuana, 10
Nardini, Norman, 162
National Enquirer, The, 147
National Highway Traffic Safety Administration, 207
National Institute of Medicine, 202
National Institute on Alcohol Abuse and Alcoholism, 207
National Institute on Drug Abuse, 201, 206
National Organization for the Reform of Marijuana Laws (NORML), 24, 170, 178, 179, 194–195
nausea, 67

Nayak, Fulla, 72, 215
Nelson, Willie, 163, 207
Netherlands, 170–171
New Riders of the Purple Sage, 159, 161
New York Academy of Medicine, 213
New York Times, 193
Nimbin, Australia, 172
Nine to Five, 144
Nixon, Richard, 207, 214
NORML Women's Alliance, 194–195
notes, tasting, 10, 12
Nurse Jackie (Showtime), 154
nutrients, growing and, 87
Nyro, Laura, 161

O

Oaksterdam University, 49, 185–186
Obama, Barack, 207
obstetrics and gynecology, 62–63
odor control, 20, 46
"One Draw," 164
one hitters, 21, 23
"One Toke Over the Line," 159
Oregon Medical Marijuana Program, 170, 179
organic, 80
organizations, 194–195
O'Shaughnessy, William, 212, 214
osteoporosis, 63

outdoor growing, 82–83
overdosing, 111–112
ovulation, human, 122

P

Pa'ia, Maui, 172
pain, 67
Palin, Sarah, 207
Panama Red, 203
"Panama Red" (New Riders of the Purple Sage), 159
Paré, Jessica, 152
parenting, 125–131
Parker, Mary-Louise, 153
parties, 133, 135–136
Parton, Dolly, 144
"Pass It, Pass It," 164
"Pass the Dutchie," 163
"Pass the Kouchie," 163
patent 6,630,507, 64, 208
Peace, Love, and Misunderstanding, 146
Peel, David, & The Lower East Side, 161
personal searches, 54
pesticides, 8–9
pests, growing and, 83, 87
petitions, 193
pets, 69
Phelps, Michael, 207
Phish, 159
Phoenix Tears, 34, 37
Pink Floyd, 159
pinner, 18
pipe pokers, 138–139

pipes, 19, 21
    buying, 23
    cleaning, 136–139
    improvised, 139, 141
Pitt, Brad, 155
"Planet of Weed," 163
plant anatomy, 12
plant gender, 85, 87
"Play the Greed," 159
pokers, 23
police encounters, 49–57
pop culture, 143–167
Popular Mechanics, 213
portable grow tents, 85
Portland Hempstalk, 176
pot party mix, 134
potency
    history of, 203–204
    testing for, 103
power outages, 84
POWs, 193–194
pre-roll, 18
Prepon, Laura, 154
Presley, Angaleena, 165
Price, April, 172
Price, Sammy, and His Texas Bluesmusicians, 156
probable cause, 51
procuring marijuana, 39–47
prohibition, origins of, 57
Psychology Today, 121–122
puff, puff, pass, 25
Purchase, Erin, 128–129, 131
purged, 34

R

Raber, Jeffrey, 8–9, 10, 37
racism, law enforcement and, 193
"Rainy Day Women # 12 and 35," 161
Ramesses II, 68, 212
Rayburn, Sam, 57
Reagan, Nancy, 151
rebuttals, challenges and, 199–211
recipes, 77, 106–107, 114–115, 123, 134
"Reefer Blues," 164
"Reefer Head Woman," 167
Reefer Madness, 143
"Reefer Man," 155
Rees, Daniel, 209
reform travel vacations, 179
Reiman, Amanda, 202
representation, legal, 53
representatives, elected, 193
reproduction, human, 122
Reynolds, John Russell, 212
rheumatoid arthritis, 63
Rhino Records, 162
Rick Simpson Oil (RSO), 34, 37
rights, legal, 49–57
Rihanna, 2, 166, 189, 207
Rivers, Joan, 155
roach paper art, 137
roaches, 19
Roberts, Julia, 144
Rogie, S. E., 163

"Roll Another Number (for the Road)," 164
"Roll Me Up," 163
rolling a joint, 16, *17*
Rolling Stone, 155, 167
Rolling Stones, 164
Romans, James, 197
Rossom, Emmy, 152
Royal Botanical Gardens, 212
Run from the Cure, 37
running, 19
Russell, Robert, 68

S

"Safe in My Garden," 156
Sagal, Katey, 152
Sagan, Carl, 207
"San Diego Reggaefornia," 163
San Diego State University, study at, 204
Sarandon, Susan, 48, 144, 147, 207
Savages, 146
schools and universities, marijuana studies in, 185–187
schwag, 5, 7, 12
scissors, 93
screens, 23
searches, 50–52, 55, 56
Seattle Hempfest, 176
security issues, 88–89
seeds, 12, 80
sex, 117–123
shake, 7

Shameless (Showtime), 152
shatter, 34
Shen Neng, 212
short order cannabis cooking, 112
shotgunning, 119, 121
side effects, 5, 99
silence, legal right to, 51, 53
Silverman, Sarah, 155, 175, 215
Simpson, Rick, 37
Sinclair, John, 176
sinsemilla, 7, 80
Six Feet Under (HBO), 153–154
Sixth Amendment, 197
skin care, 75
sleep apnea, 69
slow cookers, 105
smell control, 20, 46
Smith, Patti, 166
"Smoke a Little Smoke," 165
Smoke Buddy, 20
"Smoke Two Joints," 162
smoking etiquette, 25
smoking them out, 41
sneak-a-tokes, 21
Snoop Dogg, 155, 164
social clubs, 179
soil, 80
Sons of Anarchy (FX), 152
space, growing and, 84
spas, 77
sperm counts, human, 122
"Spinich Song, The (I Didn't Like It the First Time)," 156
spliff, 19
spoof, 20

Stafford, Jim, 162

stash, 19

storing of, 141

Stealing Beauty, 144

stealth pipes, 21

Stealth Products, 46

stems, 12

Stepmom, 144

Stewart, Jon, 207

Stewart, Kristin, 147

Stewart, Martha, 136, 155, 207, 215

Stone, Joss, 166

Stone, Oliver, 207

stone pipes, 21

"Stoned Soul Picnic," 161

stoner bands, 159

straining, cooking and, 107–108

strains, 6–7

Streisand, Barbara, 167

Students for Sensible Drug Policy (SSDP), 195

studies, evaluation of, 211

Sublime, 159, 162, 164–165

Substance Abuse and Mental Health Services Administration, 203

sugar leaves, 12

suicide rates, 204

Super High Me, 155

"Sweet Leaf," 161

"Sweet Marijuana," 156

Swerdlow, Lanny, 203

T

t-shirts, 195

"Take a Toke," 167

talking points, 199–211

Tashkin, Donald, 27, 210, 211

tasting notes, 10, 12

tasting parties, 133, 135–136

Taylor-Young, Leigh, 143

television, marijuana on, 151–154

Thai Sticks, 203

That '70s Show (Fox), 154

"That Cat Is High," 156

THC content, 203–204

theft, by police, 52

Theron, Charlize, 147

THX (Delta-9-tetrahydrocannabinol), 7, 9

thyroid problems, 63

tinctures, 34, 111

"To Be Young (Is to Be Sad, Is to Be High)," 165

Today show, 155

Toklas, Alice B., 108

Tomlin, Lily, 144, 147

Tosh, Peter, 158

tourism industry, 178–179

Toyes, 158

Traffic (band), 163

traffic accidents, surveys of, 208–209

traffic stops, 55–56

Transportation Security Administration (TSA), 169–170

transporting marijuana, 46

travel, 169–179

best locations, 170–172

expos and festivals, 172, 175–176, 178

reform efforts and, 179

tourism industry and, 178–179

trichomes, 12

trimming, 90, 93–94

Trudeau, Margaret, 214

tube style vapes, 26–27

tubular pipes, 139

Turner, Ted, 207

Turner, William, 212

Tvert, Mason, 200

"Two Hits and the Joint Turned Brown," 159

Tyler, Liv, 144

U

undercover cops, 41

United Nations, 213, 214

University of Buffalo's Research Institute on Addictions, 206

University of California at Los Angeles (UCLA), study at, 27, 210, 211

University of California at San Diego, study at, 202, 206

University of Colorado, study at, 204

University of Iowa, study at, 122

University of Sydney, study at, 72

University of Virginia, study at, 62
U.S. Constitution, 50–53, 57
U.S. government patent 6,630,507, 64, 208

V

vape pens, 26
vaporizer bags, 138
vaporizers, 20, 23
vaporizing (vaping), 24, 26–28
vegan, 80
vegetative state, 80
Victoria, Queen, 68
violence, studies on, 206
visual extravangana movies, 149–150
Volcano Brand, 28, 138
vomiting, relief from, 67
vulnerability, growing and, 83

W

Wahshiyah, Ibn, 212

Waiting to Inhale: Marijuana, Medicine and the Law, 151
"War on Drugs," 214, 215
warrants, 51–52, 56
water, growing and, 87
water hash, 32
Waters, Muddy, 164
weather, 83, 95
"Weed Instead of Roses," 167
"Weed with Willie," 159
Weeds (Showtime), 153
Weezer, 165
weight conversions, 171
Wells, Dawn, 155
Werc Shop, 8–9, 10, 37
What I Got," 164–165
What If Cannabis Cured Cancer?, 8, 127, 151
What Women Want, 146
White, Betty, 155
"Wildwood Weed," 161–162
Williams, Dar, 159

Williams, Hank, Jr., 164
Williams, Pharrell, 164
"Willin," 164
Willy Wonka and the Chocolate Factory, 149
withdrawal, 202–203
Wizard of Oz, The, 149
women musicians, cannabis and, 166
Wood, Natalie, 143
wood pipes, 21, 138
World Health Organization (WHO), 111, 206

X

xerostomia (cotton mouth), 121

Y

Yes, 159
yoga, 73, 75
Young, Francis, 200
Young, Neil, 164

PHOTO LIST

page iii: illustration by Erin Seaward-Hiatt

page vi: © istockphoto.com

page 3: © Andrew McLeod/TrunkArchive.com

page 4: © istockphoto.com

page 8: (left and right) © 123rf.com

page 9: (left and right): © 123rf.com

page 11: istockphoto.com

page 13: © bigstockphoto.com

page 14: veer.com

page 17: illlustration by Tim McGrath

page 18: © bigstockphoto.com

page 22: istockphoto.com

page 23: courtesy of KushKrystals, Etsy

page 25: © Silver Screen Collection/ MoviePix/Getty Images

page 27: © bigstockphoto.com

page 28: © 123rf.com

page 29: © 123rf.com

page 30: © DonGoofy/Flickr, https:// www.flickr.com/photos/100651935@ N07/9590486104/

page 33: © Andre Rodriquez/Flickr, https:// www.flickr.com/photos/symic/8140469407

page 36: © Nickel Bag of Funk/ Flickr, https://www.flickr.com/photos/ nickel_bag_of_funk/3487536507

page 38: istockphoto.com

page 42: © Jamie Forde/NurPhoto/ NurPhoto/Corbis

page 45: © istockphoto.com

page 47: © fotalia.com

page 48: © fotalia.com

page 51: © dreamstime.com

page 55: © dreamstime.com

page 57: © commons.wikimeida.org

page 58: © dreamstime.com

page 61: © Lew Robertson/Corbis

page 65: © istockphoto.com

page 68: © commons.wikimeida.org

page 69: © 123rf.com

page 70: © 123rf.com

page 74: © shutterstock

page 76: courtesy of Dr. Bronner's Magic Soaps

page 78: © istockphoto.com

page 81: © 123rf.com

page 86: © istockphoto.com

page 91: © Naberacka/Flickr, https://www. flickr.com/photos/naberacka/9213637067

page 92: © Mark/Flickr, https://www.flickr. com/photos/eggrole/4982293716/

page 96: © veer.com

page 101: © 123rf.com

page 106: © 123rf.com

page 107: © istockphoto.com

page 108: © 123rf.com

page 113: © istockphoto.com

page 116: © 123rf.com

page 120: © istockphoto.com

page 124: © fotalia.com

page 127: © 123rf.com

page 129: © rObz/flickr, https://www.flickr. com/photos/acci0n/128657844/

page 132: © fotalia.com

page 135: © dreamstime.com

page 140: © Cheri Sicard

page 142: © canstockphoto.com

page 145: © Mondadori/Getty Images

page 148: © canstockphoto.com

page 153: (sofa image) © canstockphoto.com; (marijuana leaf on tv) © 123rf.com

page 157: (turntable) © canstockphoto.com; (marijuana leaf) © 123rf.com

page 160: © canstockphoto.com

page 167: © 123rf.com

page 168: © Iain Masterton/Alamy

page 173: © istockphoto.com

page 174: © istockphoto.com

page 177: © 123rf.com

page 180: © istockphoto.com

page 183: © fotalia.com

page 186: courtesy of Oaksterdam University

page 187: courtesy of Oaksterdam University

page 188: © Target Presse Agentur Gmbh/ Getty Images Entertainment

page 192: © fotalia.com

page 196: courtesy Lisa Koluvek of Beastly Luck

page 198: (bull's eye) © bigstockphoto.com; (marijuana leaf) © 123rf.com

page 205: © 123rf.com

page 210: © 123rf.com

page 216: © 123rf.com

page 232: © 123rf.com

REFERENCE LIST

STUDIES AND REPORTS

Tashkin, Donald P. "Effects of Marijuana Smoking on the Lung." Annals of the American Thoracic Society, Vol. 10, No. 3. 2013.

Gieringer, Dale; St. Laurent, Joseph; Goodrich, Scott. "Cannabis Vaporizer Combines Efficient Delivery of THC with Effective Suppression of Pyrolytic Compounds." Journal of Cannabis Therapeutics, Vol. 4(1) 2004.

Elizabeth A. Penner, MD, MPH; Hannah Buettner, BA; Murray A. Mittleman, MD, DrPH. "The Impact of Marijuana Use on Glucose, Insulin, and Insulin Resistance among US Adults." American Journal of Medicine 2013.

Dreher, Melanie C.; Nugent, Kevin;, Hudgins, Rebekah. "Prenatal Marijuana Exposure and Neonatal Outcomes in Jamaica: An Ethnographic Study." Journal of the American Academy of Pediatrics 1992.

Liang C, McClean MD, Marsit C, Christensen B, Peters E, Nelson HH, Kelsey KT. "A population-based case-control study of marijuana use and head and neck squamous cell carcinoma." National Institutes of Health 2009.

Appendino G; Gibbons S; Giana A; Pagani A; Grassi G; Stavri M; Smith E; Rahman MM. "Antibacterial cannabinoids from Cannabis sativa: a structure-activity study." National Institutes of Health 2008.

Block, R.I. et al. "Effects of Chronic Marijuana Use on Testosterone, Luteinizing Hormone, Follicle Stimulating Hormone, Prolactin and Cortisol in Men and Women," Drug and Alcohol Dependence 28:121–8 (1991).

Degenhardt, L., L. Dierker, W. T. Chiu, M. E. Medina-Mora, Y. Neumark, N. Sampson, J. Alonso, et al. "Evaluating the Drug Use "Gateway" Theory Using Cross-National Data: Consistency and Associations of the Order of Initiation of Drug Use among Participants in the Who World Mental Health Surveys."

Jacobus, J. et al. "White matter integrity in adolescents with histories of marijuana use and binge drinking." Neurotoxicology and Teratology. Volume 31, Issue 6, November–December 2009.

Joy, Janet E; Watson, Stanley J, Jr.; Benson, John A, Jr.; editors. "Marijuana and Medicine:

Assessing the Science Base." National Academy of Sciences' Institute of Medicine 1999.

Anderson, D. Mark; Rees, Daniel I; Sabia, Joseph, J. "High on Life: Medical Marijuana Laws and Suicide." The Institute for the Study of Labor (IZA) 2012.

Tait, Robert J; Mackinnon, Andrew; Christensen, Helen. "Cannabis use and cognitive function: 8-year trajectory in a young adult cohort." Society for the Study of Addiction 2011.

Anderson, D. Mark; Rees, Daniel I; "Medical Marijuana Laws, Traffic Fatalities, and Alcohol Consumption." Journal of Law and Economics 2013.

American Civil Liberties Union. "The War on Marijuana in Black and White" 2013.

Federal Bureau of Investigation. "Crime in the United States, 2012." Washington, DC: U.S. Department of Justice 2013.

BOOKS

Armentano, Paul. "Emerging Clinical Application for Cannabis and Cannabinoids: A Review of Recent Scientific Literature" (5th Edition). The NORML Foundation 2012.

Leiderman, Jay; Devine, James P. "Medical Marijuana Law in California." The NORML Foundation 2011.

Armentano, Paul; Fox, Steve; Tvert, Mason; *Marijuana is Safer: So Why Are We Driving People To Drink?* Chelsea Green Publishing; 2 edition 2013.

Werner, Clint. *Marijuana, Gateway to Health: How Cannabis Protects Us from Cancer and Alzheimer's Disease.* Dachstar Press 2011

Grinspoon, Lester, MD; Bakalar, Dr. James B. *Marijuana: The Forbidden Medicine.* Yale University Press; Revised edition 1997.

Cervantes, Jorge. *Marijuana Horticulture: he Indoor/Outdoor Medical Grower's Bible.* Van Patten Publishing; 5th edition 2006.

Rosenthal, Ed. "Marijuana Grower's Handbook: Your Complete Guide for Medical and Personal Cultivation." Quick American Archives 2010.

Stitch, JC; Rosenthal, Ed. "Marijuana Garden Saver: Handbook for Healthy Plants." Quick American Archives 2008.

Rosenthal, Ed. "Marijuana Gold: Trash to Stash." Quick American Archives 2002.

WEBSITES

All of the following websites contain a wealth of information, far too many articles and studies to cite each individually, but chances are you can find an accurate answer to any question about marijuana you might have, from medical, legal and political matters, to cultivation, lifestyle, women's issues, history, pop culture, and more at the following websites.

Drug Policy Alliance. "10 Facts About Marijuana": www.drugpolicy.org/drug-facts/10-facts-about-marijuana

ProCon.org. "Medical Marijuana Pros and Cons": medicalmarijuana.procon.org

Schaffer Library of Drug Policy: "Hemp/Marijuana": www.druglibrary.org/schaffer/hemp/hempmenu.htm

Project CBD: www.projectcbd.org

Law Enforcement Against Prohibition: www.leap.cc

National Organization for the Reform of Marijuana Laws: www.norml.org

Marijuana Policy Project: www.mpp.org

Flex Your Rights: www.flexyourrights.org

Fully Informed Jury Association: www.fija.org

High Times : www.hightimes.com

Ladybud: www.ladybud.com

Tokin' Woman: tokinwoman.blogspot.com

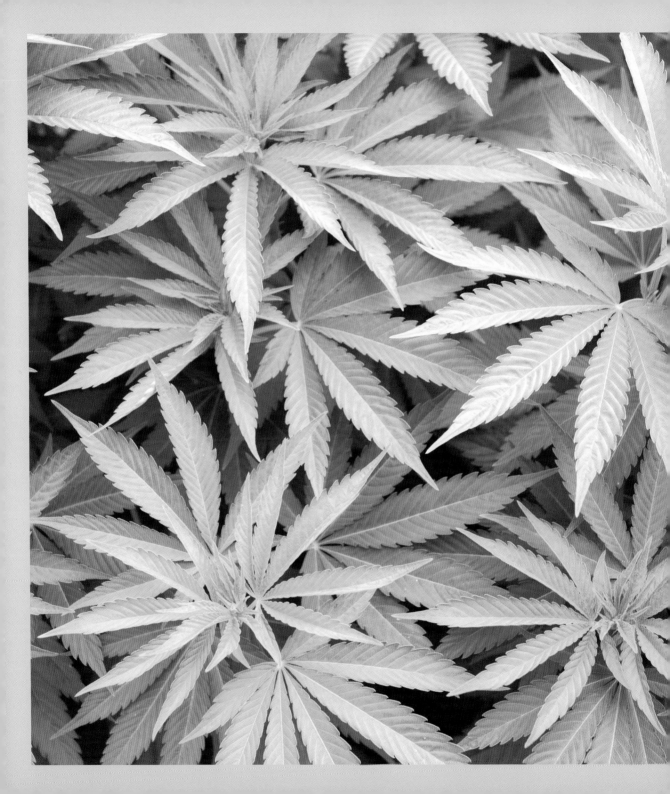

ABOUT THE AUTHOR

Cheri Sicard never would have thought that she would one day become a passionate marijuana activist. Once a closeted medical marijuana user, she now works with numerous reform groups and frequently organizes rallies, speaks at city council meetings, and gives classes on various aspects of marijuana. She also advocates for clemency on behalf of prisoners serving life sentences for nonviolent marijuana offenses.

Cheri is a professional writer, recipe developer, and internet entrepreneur. Her earlier books include *The Great American Handbook, U.S. Citizenship for Dummies,* and *Everyday American*. In addition, Cheri's Cannabis Gourmet Cookbook is one of the most popular and well-reviewed books of its kind.

SELECTED TITLES *from* SEAL PRESS

Drinking Diaries: Women Serve Their Stories Straight Up, edited by Caren Osten Gerszberg and Leah Odze Epstein. $16.00, 978-1-58005-411-9. Celebrated writers take a candid look at the pleasures and pains of drinking, and the many ways in which it touches women's lives.

Got Teens?: The Doctor Moms' Guide to Sexuality, Social Media and Other Adolescent Realities, by Logan Levkoff, PhD and Jennifer Wider, MD. $16.00, 978-1-58005-506-2. Adolescent health and sexuality experts provide parents of middle schoolers a way to decode their teen's health questions and behavior.

The Good Mother Myth: Redefining Motherhood to Fit Reality, edited by Avital Norman Nathman. $16.00, 978-1-58005-502-4. This collection of essays takes a realistic look at motherhood and provides a platform for real voices and raw stories, each offering an honest perspective on what it means to be a mother.

The New I Do: Reshaping Marriage for Skeptics, Realists, and Rebels, by Susan Pease Gadoua and Vicki Larson. $17.00, 978-1-58005-545-1. A new perspective on the modern shape of marriage, this guide offers couples a roadmap for creating alternative marital partnerships.

Better than Perfect: 7 Strategies to Crush Your Inner Critic and Create a Life You Love, by Elizabeth Lombardo. $16.00, 978-1-58005-549-9. A proven, powerful method for shaking the chains of perfectionism and finding balance in life.

Toss the Gloss: Beauty Tips, Tricks & Truths for Women 50+, by Andrea Q. Robinson. $24.00, 978-1-58005-490-4. Industry insider Andrea Q. Robinson—former beauty editor at Vogue, president of Tom Ford Beauty, and more—shares her ultimate guide to looking great at age 50 and beyond.

Find Seal Press Online
www.sealpress.com
www.facebook.com/sealpress
Twitter: @SealPress